Sleep Disorders and Psychiatry

Review of Psychiatry Series
John M. Oldham, M.D., M.S.
Michelle B. Riba, M.D., M.S.
Series Editors

Sleep Disorders and Psychiatry

EDITED BY

Daniel J. Buysse, M.D.

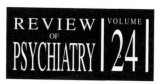

No. 2

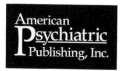

Washington, DC
London, England

Copyright © 2005 American Psychiatric Publishing, Inc.
ALL RIGHTS RESERVED

Manufactured in the United States of America on acid-free paper
08 07 06 05 04   5 4 3 2 1
First Edition

Typeset in Adobe's Palatino.

American Psychiatric Publishing, Inc.
1000 Wilson Boulevard
Arlington, VA 22209-3901
www.appi.org

The correct citation for this book is
Buysse DJ (editor): *Sleep Disorders and Psychiatry* (Review of Psychiatry Series, Volume 24, Number 2; Oldham JM and Riba MB, series editors). Washington, DC, American Psychiatric Publishing, 2005

Library of Congress Cataloging-in-Publication Data
Sleep disorders and psychiatry / edited by Daniel J. Buysse. -- 1st ed.
    p. ; cm. -- (Review of psychiatry ; v. 24, no. 2)
  Includes bibliographical references and index.
  ISBN 1-58562-229-X (pbk. : alk. paper)
  1. Sleep disorders.
  [DNLM: 1. Sleep Disorders--diagnosis. 2. Sleep Disorders--therapy. 3. Circadian Rhythm. 4. Sleep--physiology. 5. Sleep Disorders--physiopathology.]
  I. Buysse, Daniel J. II. Series: Review of psychiatry series ; v. 24, 2.

RC547.S5195 2005
61.8'498--dc22   2005002344

British Library Cataloguing in Publication Data
A CIP record is available from the British Library.

This volume is dedicated to my parents,
Jerry and Rosemary Buysse.

Contents

Contributors

Jed E. Black, M.D.
Director, Stanford Sleep Disorders Clinic; Assistant Professor, Department of Psychiatry and Behavioral Sciences, Stanford University, Stanford, California

Stephen N. Brooks, M.D.
Assistant Clinical Professor, Department of Psychiatry and Behavioral Sciences, Stanford University, Stanford, California

Daniel J. Buysse, M.D.
Professor of Psychiatry and Director, Clinical Neuroscience Research Center, Department of Psychiatry, University of Pittsburgh School of Medicine, Pittsburgh, Pennsylvania

Nilesh B. Davé, M.D., M.P.H.
Fellow, Pulmonary, Allergy, and Critical Care Medicine, University of Pittsburgh Medical Center, Pittsburgh, Pennsylvania

Anne Germain, Ph.D.
Postdoctoral Research Fellow, University of Pittsburgh School of Medicine, Pittsburgh, Pennsylvania

Prasanth Manthena, M.D.
Instructor of Neurology, Northwestern University Feinberg School of Medicine, Chicago, Illinois

Douglas Moul, M.D.
Assistant Professor of Psychiatry, University of Pittsburgh School of Medicine, Pittsburgh, Pennsylvania

Seiji Nishino, M.D., Ph.D.
Associate Professor, Department of Psychiatry and Behavioral Sciences, Stanford University, Stanford, California

Eric A. Nofzinger, M.D.
Associate Professor of Psychiatry and Director, Sleep Neuroimaging Research Program, University of Pittsburgh School of Medicine, Pittsburgh, Pennsylvania

John M. Oldham, M.D., M.S.
Professor and Chair, Department of Psychiatry and Behavioral Sciences, Medical University of South Carolina, Charleston, South Carolina

Michelle B. Riba, M.D., M.S.
Clinical Professor and Associate Chair for Education and Academic Affairs, Department of Psychiatry, University of Michigan Medical School, Ann Arbor, Michigan

Patrick J. Strollo, Jr., M.D.
Medical Director, UPMC Sleep Medicine Center; Associate Professor of Medicine, Division of Pulmonary, Allergy, and Critical Care Medicine, University of Pittsburgh School of Medicine, Pittsburgh, Pennsylvania

John W. Winkelman, M.D., Ph.D.
Medical Director, Sleep Health Center, Division of Sleep Medicine, Brigham and Women's Hospital, Boston, Massachusetts; Assistant Professor of Psychiatry, Harvard Medical School, Boston, Massachusetts

Phyllis Zee, M.D., Ph.D.
Professor of Neurology and Director, Sleep Disorders Center, Northwestern University Feinberg School of Medicine, Chicago, Illinois

Introduction to the Review of Psychiatry Series

John M. Oldham, M.D., M.S.
Michelle B. Riba, M.D., M.S.

2005 REVIEW OF PSYCHIATRY SERIES TITLES

- *Psychiatric Genetics*
  EDITED BY KENNETH S. KENDLER, M.D., AND LINDON EAVES, PH.D., D.SC.
- *Sleep Disorders and Psychiatry*
  EDITED BY DANIEL J. BUYSSE, M.D.
- *Advances in Treatment of Bipolar Disorder*
  EDITED BY TERENCE A. KETTER, M.D.
- *Mood and Anxiety Disorders During Pregnancy and Postpartum*
  EDITED BY LEE S. COHEN, M.D., AND RUTA M. NONACS, M.D., PH.D.

The Annual Review of Psychiatry has been published for almost a quarter of a century, and 2005 marks the final year of publication of this highly successful series. First published in 1982, the Annual Review was conceived as a single volume highlighting new developments in the field that would be informative and of practical value to mental health practitioners. From the outset, the Annual Review was coordinated with the Annual Meeting of the American Psychiatric Association (APA), so that the material from each year's volume could also be presented in person by the chapter authors at the Annual Meeting. In its early years, the Review was one of a relatively small number of major books regularly published by American Psychiatric Press, Inc. (APPI; now American Psychiatric Publishing, Inc.). Through the subsequent years, however, the demand for new authoritative material led to an exponential growth in the number of new titles published by APPI each year. New published material became more readily available throughout each year, so that the unique function originally provided by the Annual Review was no longer needed.

Times change in many ways. The increased production volume, depth, and diversity of APPI's timely and authoritative material, now rapidly being augmented by electronic publishing, are welcome changes, and it is appropriate that this year's volume of the Annual Review represents the final curtain of the series. We have been privileged to be coeditors of the Annual Review for over a decade, and we are proud to have been a part of this distinguished series.

We hope you will agree that Volume 24 wonderfully lives up to the traditionally high standards of the Annual Review. In *Psychiatric Genetics*, edited by Kendler and Eaves, the fast-breaking and complex world of the genetics of psychiatric disorders is addressed. Following Kendler's clear and insightful introductory overview, Eaves, Chen, Neale, Maes, and Silberg present a careful analysis of the various methodologies used today to study the genetics of complex diseases in human populations. In turn, the book presents the latest findings on the genetics of schizophrenia, by Riley and Kendler; of anxiety disorders, by Hettema; of substance use disorders, by Prescott, Maes, and Kendler; and of antisocial behavior, by Jacobson.

Sleep Disorders and Psychiatry, edited by Buysse, brings us up to date on the sleep disorders from a psychiatric perspective, reviewing critically important clinical conditions that may not always receive the priority they deserve. Following a comprehensive introductory chapter, Buysse then presents, with his colleagues Germain, Moul, and Nofzinger, an authoritative review of the fundamental and pervasive problem of insomnia. Strollo and Davé next review sleep apnea, a potentially life-threatening condition that can also be an unrecognized source of excessive daytime sleepiness and impaired functioning. Black, Nishino, and Brooks present the basics of narcolepsy, along with new findings and treatment recommendations. In two separate chapters, Winkelman then reviews the parasomnias and the particular problem of restless legs syndrome. The book concludes with an extremely important chapter by Zee and Manthena reviewing circadian rhythm sleep disorders.

Advances in Treatment of Bipolar Disorder, edited by Ketter, provides an update on bipolar disorder. Following an introductory overview by Ketter, Sachs, Bowden, Calabrese, Chang, and Rasgon on the advances in the treatment of bipolar disorder, more specific material is presented on the treatment of acute mania, by Ketter, Wang, Nowakowska, Marsh, and Bonner. Sachs then presents a current look at the treatment of acute depression in bipolar patients, followed by a review by Bowden and Singh of the long-term management of bipolar disorder. The problem of rapid cycling is taken up by Muzina, Elhaj, Gajwani, Gao, and Calabrese. Chang, Howe, and Simeonova then discuss the treatment of children and adolescents with bipolar disorder, and the concluding chapter, by Rasgon and Zappert, provides a special focus on women with bipolar disorder.

Mood and Anxiety Disorders During Pregnancy and Postpartum, edited by Cohen and Nonacs, concerns the range of issues of psychiatric relevance related to pregnancy and the postpartum period. Cohen and Nonacs review the course of psychiatric illness during pregnancy, and the postpartum period is covered by Petrillo, Nonacs, Viguera, and Cohen. In this review, the authors focus particularly on depression, bipolar disorder, anxiety disorders, and psychotic disorders. The diagnosis and treatment of mood and anxiety disorders during pregnancy are then discussed in more detail in the subsequent chapter by Nonacs, Cohen, Viguera, and Mogielnicki, followed by a more in-depth look at management of bipolar disorder by Viguera, Cohen, Nonacs, and Baldessarini. Nonacs then presents a comprehensive and important look at the postpartum period, concentrating on mood disorders. This chapter is followed by a discussion of the use of antidepressants and mood-stabilizing medications during breast-feeding, by Ragan, Stowe, and Newport. Overall, this book provides up-to-date information about the management of common psychiatric disorders during gestation and during the critical postpartum period.

Before closing this final version of our annual introductory comments, we would like to thank all of the authors who have contributed so generously to the Annual Review, as well as the editors who preceded us. In addition, we thank the wonderful staff at APPI who have so diligently helped produce a quality product each year, and we would particularly like to thank our two administrative assistants, Liz Bednarowicz and Linda Gacioch, without whom the work could not have been done.

Acknowledgments

Editing this volume has led to more sleeplessness—and more satisfaction—than I would have first guessed. But I have shared both the challenges and the rewards, and acknowledgments are due to many people.

First, I wish to thank the authors and co-authors of chapters in this volume for sharing their knowledge and clinical wisdom. It was a pleasure to work with such talented writers and educators, and to do so with a minimum of cajoling.

Second, thanks to the staff at the University of Pittsburgh, particularly Melissa Shablesky, who helped whip everything into shape, including the many tricky figures you see in this volume.

Third, thanks to John Oldham and his staff for using their experience to guide everyone else through the writing process, and to the staff of American Psychiatric Publishing, Inc., for working efficiently through production.

Fourth, I would like to thank my friends and colleagues at the University of Pittsburgh and throughout the field of sleep medicine. You have taught me and inspired me and have proven that diversity leads to strength.

Finally, and most important, I wish to thank my family—Sandy, Caitlin, Allison, and Evan—for putting up with longer hours and more travel than is reasonable. Your love and support are the things that dreams are made of.

Chapter 1

Introduction

Daniel J. Buysse, M.D.

Sleep and wakefulness are fundamental behavioral and neurobiological states that characterize all higher animals, including human beings. Indeed, the universal nature of sleep-wake states and their rhythmic occurrence are so elementary that it is easy to overlook their salience for mental health, physical health, and functioning.

Although the function of sleep and sleep-wake rhythms has long been debated, it is unlikely that such a fundamental process will ever be equated with one single function. Just as one never questions the "function" of wakefulness, the functions of sleep may be so intrinsic to higher biological systems that they elude simple description. Several major theories of the function of sleep and sleep-wake rhythms include the following:

- *Ecological or environmental advantage.* Sleep provides a regular period of behavioral inactivity that may help to match animals to their ideal environmental situation. For example, for human beings, with their strong reliance on vision, wakefulness during daylight makes evolutionary "sense"; rodents such as rats and mice, who rely more on touch and smell, may be better adapted to be awake during the dark period and asleep during the light period. The hypothesis of environmental advantage is supported by a study of normally day-active chipmunks with surgical lesions of the biological clock. Compared with control animals, lesioned chipmunks had greater nighttime activity

Work on this chapter was supported by National Institutes of Health grants MH24652, AG00972, AG20677, and RR00056.

and higher mortality due to weasel predation when reintroduced to their natural environment (DeCoursey et al. 2000).

- *"Physical restoration."* It was once thought that protein metabolism is in a more anabolic state during sleep than during wakefulness. However, quiet wakefulness achieves much the same effect as actual sleep in terms of such effects. It has been noted that sleep deprivation is associated with impaired glucose metabolism and relative insulin insensitivity (Spiegel et al. 1999). Sleep deprivation is also associated with altered measures of immune function (Spiegel et al. 2002), suggesting that sleep may play important host defense roles as well.

- *Optimizing waking function.* Studies indicate that sleep deprivation in humans and animals is associated with clear decrements in subjective alertness, vigilance, and decision making (Belenky et al. 2003; Harrison and Horne 2000; VanDongen et al. 2003). In addition, sleep deprivation has adverse effects on mood (Pilcher and Huffcutt 1996). Thus, one of sleep's important functions may be to preserve and optimize waking brain function.

- *Learning and integration of experience.* Visual and other forms of learning are enhanced by sleep and are impaired by sleep loss (Stickgold et al. 2000). In addition, rapid eye movement (REM) sleep is associated with activation of limbic system structures, suggesting a role in emotional processing (Nofzinger et al. 1997). Thus, sleep may affect not only cognitive function, but also the ability to accumulate experience and to learn—both in cognitive and affective domains.

- *Survival.* Studies in rats show that death is the inevitable consequence of prolonged sleep deprivation (Rechtschaffen et al. 1989). In human beings, epidemiologic studies have shown an association between extremes of sleep duration and mortality; both short (<5 hours) and long (>9 hours) sleep durations are associated with greater risk (Kripke et al. 2002). Disorders of sleep also have clear adverse consequences for health outcomes. For instance, insomnia is clearly associated with increased risk for subsequent depression (Riemann and Voderholzer 2003), obstructive sleep apnea syndrome is associated with increased risk of subsequent cardiovascular disease and hypertension (Peppard et al. 2000), and REM sleep behavior disorder is associated with increased development of Lewy body disease (Turner 2002). Conversely, virtually every psychiatric disorder and a wide variety of medical illnesses adversely affect sleep. Therefore, sleep is essential for good health, and health, in turn, affects sleep.

Neurobiology of Circadian Rhythms

The sleep-wake cycle is the most obvious of the 24-hour (circadian) rhythms that govern most physiological systems (Czeisler and Khalsa 2000) (see Chapter 7, "Circadian Rhythm Sleep Disorders," in this volume). Biological rhythms can have many different *periods* (i.e., the time to complete one cycle). For instance, electroencephalographic (EEG) and cardiac rhythms occur with a period, and on the order, of seconds or fractions of a second; sleep-wake stages cycle with periods of 1–2 hours, exemplifying ultradian rhythms; the sleep-wake rhythm itself cycles with a 24-hour rhythm, an example of a circadian rhythm; and other rhythms, such as menstrual and hibernation rhythms, have much longer periods (infradian rhythms). The *amplitude* of rhythm is a measure of the "size" of oscillation and is technically defined as one-half of the peak/trough difference. *Phase* refers to the timing of a rhythm relative to some reference point such as clock time, onset of the light portion of the day, or another biological rhythm. Virtually all physiological systems in humans show circadian variation, including endocrine rhythms such as cortisol and melatonin, core body temperature, and urine volume. Furthermore, cognitive and performance variables also show circadian variation, including measures such as subjective sleepiness and alertness, reaction time, and cognitive throughput.

Circadian rhythms are *endogenous* (i.e., inherent) properties of mammalian physiology. Although circadian rhythms are often synchronized to external time cues, they continue to be expressed independent of these cues, as evidenced by experiments conducted under conditions of time isolation. *Entrainment* is the process by which endogenous rhythms are synchronized to the environment. Environmental time cues are often referred to as *zeitgebers,* or time givers. *Masking* refers to the effects of environmental or behavioral stimuli to change the appearance of an endogenous rhythm. For instance, sleep at night exerts a masking effect on core body temperature rhythms by increasing the amplitude; although core body temperature continues to have a circadian rhythm in individuals who are awake for 24 hours or longer, the amplitude is diminished in the absence of sleep. On the other hand, sleep does not exert a masking effect on the circadian rhythm of melatonin, which is present whether the individual is awake or asleep, but light shows a strong masking effect, completely suppressing melatonin secretion.

Human beings are now known to have an endogenous circadian rhythm period of just over 24 hours (Czeisler et al. 1999). In human beings and most mammals, light is the strongest zeitgeber for entraining circadian rhythms. However, the effect of zeitgebers is time dependent. For instance, bright light given toward the end of the natural sleep period in humans causes circadian rhythms to move to an earlier time ("phase advance"), whereas light given near the time of usual bedtime causes circadian rhythms to move to a later time (" phase delay").

Circadian rhythms are generated and controlled within the central nervous system. The master pacemaker of the circadian system resides in the paired suprachiasmatic nuclei (SCN) of the hypothalamus, which are located at the base of the third ventricle just above the optic chiasm. These small paired nuclei receive direct photic input from specialized ganglion cells in the retina, which travel via the retinohypothalamic tract to the SCN. The SCN has efferent pathways to the hypothalamus and thalamus, through which it transmits timing information to the rest of the central nervous system (Czeisler and Khalsa 2000; Pace-Schott and Hobson 2002). Recent developments have shown that the basis of circadian rhythmicity is a transcription-translation feedback loop involving a set of approximately nine circadian genes (King and Takahashi 2000). These genes code for protein products that have feedback control over their own production, cycling on a near 24-hour rhythm. Animals with mutations in clock genes have periods that are very short or very long compared with those of wild animals. In humans, too, genetic variation is associated with abnormal circadian rhythm phases (see Chapter 7, "Circadian Rhythm Sleep Disorders").

Sleep and Wakefulness

Sleep is a periodic, rapidly reversible neurobehavioral state characterized by almost simultaneous change in the activity patterns and mode of firing of central nervous system neurons and circuits. Periodicity is the most dominant feature of human circadian rhythms. Rapid reversibility distinguishes sleep from pathological states such as coma and unconsciousness. Nevertheless, sleep itself is an involuntary process that occurs only when proper environmental and internal circumstances are present.

In humans, characteristics of sleep are typically studied by polysomnography (PSG), an adaptation of electroencephalography. A polysomnogram includes at least one channel of EEG measurement, typically from a central lead; an electrooculographic (EOG) recording to measure eye movements; and an electromyographic (EMG) recording to measure muscle tone, typically in the submentalis muscles. The pattern of EEG activity, eye movements, and muscle tone reveal clear differences between wakefulness and sleep, which can be further divided into REM sleep and non-REM (NREM) sleep. Wakefulness, REM sleep, and NREM sleep are the three normally occurring neurobehavioral states in humans (Carskadon and Dement 2000). Each of these three states is distinguished by characteristic patterns of environmental responsiveness, general physiology, EEG waveforms, muscle tone, and mental activity. A brief comparison of these three states is presented in Table 1–1. NREM sleep is further divided into four stages of increasing "depth," which coincide with decreasing arousability. Thus, Stage 1 NREM sleep is a transitional sleep stage, Stage 2 occupies most of NREM sleep, and Stages 3 and 4 are "deep" NREM sleep, also referred to as slow-wave sleep or delta sleep because the predominant EEG pattern is one of slow (delta) activity. Examples of polysomnographic patterns in the different stages of sleep are shown in Figure 1–1.

Table 1–1. Physiological characteristics of sleep-wake states

Measure	Wake	NREM	REM
EEG	Fast, low voltage	Slow, high voltage	Fast, low voltage
Eye movement	Vision related	Slow irregular	Rapid
Neuronal activity			
In LDT/PPT	+	0	++
In LC/DR/TMN	++	+	0
In VLPO (cluster)	0	++	+?
In VLPO (extended)	0	+?	++
In hypocretin neurons	++	0?	0
Muscle tone	++	+	0
Heart rate, blood pressure, respiratory rate	Variable	Slow / low, regular	Variable, higher than NREM
Responses to hypoxia and hypercarbia	Active	Reduced responsiveness	Lowest responsiveness
Thermoregulation	Behavioral and physiological regulation	Physiological regulation only	Reduced physiological regulation
Mental activity	Full	None or limited	Story-like dreams

Note. REM=rapid eye movement sleep; NREM=non-REM sleep; EEG=electroencephalogram; LDT=laterodorsal pontine tegmentum; PPT=pedunculopontine tegmentum; LC=locus coeruleus; DR=dorsal raphe; TMN=tuberomamillary nucleus; VLPO (cluster)=central portion of ventrolateral preoptic nucleus; VLPO (extended)=peripheral portion of ventrolateral preoptic nucleus. +=activity level; 0=inactive.

Source. Adapted from Saper et al. 2001.

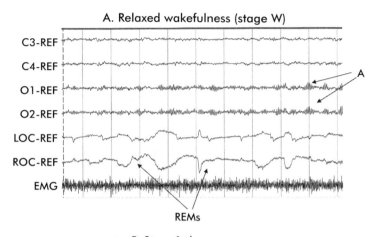

A. Relaxed wakefulness (stage W)

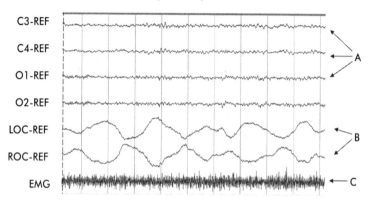

B. Stage 1 sleep

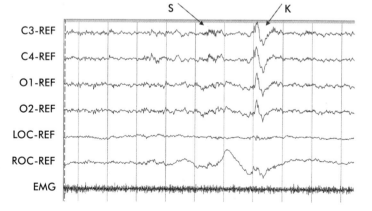

C. Stage 2 sleep

D. Stage 3 sleep

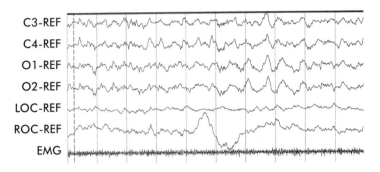

E. Stage 4 sleep

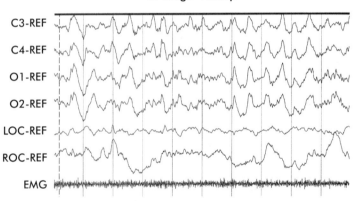

F. Rapid eye movement (REM) sleep

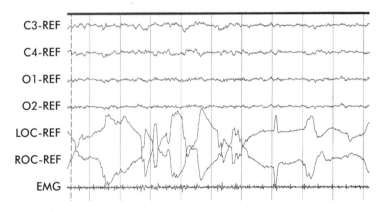

Figure 1–1. Polysomnography in different sleep stages.

The six panels show activity in the electroencephalographic (EEG), electrooculographic (EOG), and electromyographic (EMG) patterns during wakefulness and the different sleep stages. Each tracing shows 30 seconds. **A:** Wakefulness is characterized by a low-voltage, fast-frequency EEG pattern, voluntary eye movements, and tonic muscle tone. The EEG segments marked "A" show alpha rhythm, which is characteristic of relaxed wakefulness with eyes closed. The arrows marked "REMs" show rapid eye movements. The channels are labeled on the left side: C3, C4, O1, and O2 are EEG leads, which are measured relative to a common, or referential (REF), lead. LOC and ROC are leads at the left and right outer canthus of the eye. **B:** Stage 1 non-REM (NREM) sleep is characterized by a slight increase in EEG amplitude and slowing of EEG frequencies (A), slow rolling eye movements, indicated by reciprocal "hills and valleys" in the EOG channels (B), and lower muscle tone (C). **C:** Stage 2 NREM sleep is characterized by further slowing of the EEG frequencies, together with an increase in amplitude. Phasic events include "K complexes," isolated large-amplitude slow EEG waves (K); and "sleep spindles" (S), episodic bursts of fast EEG activity lasting approximately 0.5 seconds. EOG tracing shows underlying brain electrical activity, and therefore resembles the EEG pattern. Muscle tone is further reduced. **D:** Stage 3 sleep is characterized by large-amplitude, slow (0.5 – 4.0 Hz) EEG activity, also known as "delta" or "slow-wave sleep" activity, that constitutes 20%–50% of the 30-second epoch. EOG pattern mirrors EEG activity, and muscle tone is low. **E:** Stage 4 sleep is identical to Stage 3, except that delta activity occupies greater than 50% of the epoch. **F:** REM sleep is characterized by the return of faster-frequency, mixed-voltage EEG pattern, similar to Stage 1 NREM sleep. The hallmark of REM is the appearance of phasic rapid eye movements, which present as large-amplitude, "spiky" waveforms that clearly differ from the slower eye movements of Stage 1 NREM. Muscle tone is essentially absent, except for the intermittent occurrence of phasic muscle twitches, which often accompany eye movements.

In human studies, the polysomnogram is typically "scored" by a human reviewer as wakefulness, REM, or one of the four NREM sleep stages for every 30-second epoch of recording. When successive 30-second epochs are diagrammed, the result is a sleep *histogram* or *hypnogram* as displayed in Figure 1–2. This figure reveals several important aspects of normal human adult sleep. First, human beings enter sleep through light NREM sleep stages, followed by progressively deeper NREM sleep stages. Second, most of the Stage 3 and 4 or "deep" NREM sleep occurs in the first half of the night. Stage 3/4 sleep is the portion of sleep that the brain recovers following sleep deprivation. Third, NREM and REM sleep alternate approximately every 90–100 minutes during the night. Finally, REM sleep episodes tend to

A. Young adult

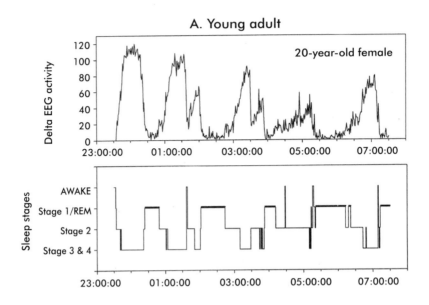

B. Older adult

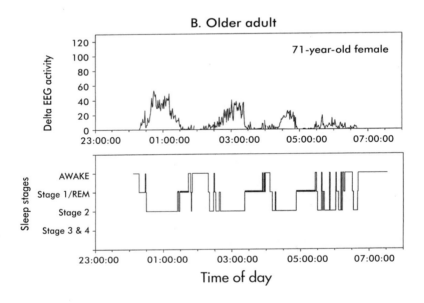

Time of day

Figure 1–2. Hypnograms and delta electroencephalographic (EEG) activity in healthy subjects.

Each 20–30-second epoch of sleep for an entire night is assigned a sleep stage by a human scorer. These epoch scores can then be displayed graphically in a "hypnogram" to display the progression of sleep stages across the night. **A:** Hypnogram (lower panel) for an entire night of sleep in a healthy young adult. Sleep stages are indicated by increasing depth on the vertical axis, with rapid eye movement (REM) sleep represented by heavy horizontal lines. Time is indicated on the horizontal axis. Note that most Stage 3/4 non-REM (NREM) sleep occurs in the early part of the night and that REM periods get longer toward the end of the night. The time course of EEG delta activity, determined by computer algorithm, is shown in the upper panel. Note that the greatest amount of delta activity (highest "peaks") occurs early in the night (roughly corresponding to Stages 3 and 4), with decreasing amounts toward the end of the night. Very little delta activity occurs during REM sleep. **B:** Hypnogram (lower panel) and EEG delta activity (upper panel) for an older adult. Note the absence of Stage 3/4 NREM sleep, the decrease in delta activity, and the greater amount of wakefulness during the sleep period.

become longer and more intense (as measured by the number of eye movements and complexity of dream mentation) toward the morning wake hours, in contrast to NREM sleep. Figure 1–2 also shows computer-generated measures of EEG delta waves during NREM sleep. These additional panels show the decrease in delta activity during the course of the night.

EEG sleep stages are normally affected by subject and environmental factors. Most important, age has prominent effects on sleep stages (see Figure 1–2). Across the adult lifespan, Stage 3 and 4 sleep gradually diminish from their peak in late adolescent years. In later adulthood, the number and the duration of awakenings during sleep increase, and the amount of Stage 1 sleep also increases. Stage 2 NREM and REM sleep are relatively consistent in amount across the adult lifespan. In addition, the entire sleep period tends to delay (occur at a later time) during adolescence, then to advance (occur at an earlier time) during later adulthood. A wide variety of sleep disorders and medication effects can influence sleep, as discussed in subsequent chapters of this volume.

Human sleep is physiologically regulated by two processes, a homeostatic factor and a circadian factor (Figure 1–3). The homeostatic factor represents an increase in sleep "drive" as a func-

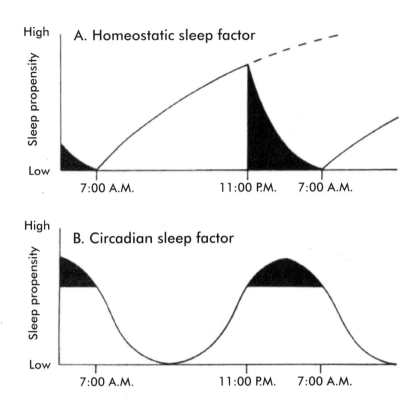

Figure 1–3. Two-process model of sleep regulation in humans.
A: The homeostatic sleep factor describes the increasing sleep drive, or sleep propensity, that occurs with increasing duration of wakefulness. The curving line represents this increasing sleep drive. The vertical axis represents sleep propensity, and the horizontal axis represents time. Sleep drive increases with progressive wakefulness, then diminishes during subsequent sleep (indicated by the black area). Homeostatic sleep drive is proportional to the amount of electroencephalographic (EEG) delta activity during sleep and the amount of EEG theta activity during wakefulness. **B:** The circadian sleep factor is driven by the biological clock. Circadian sleep drive varies with a 24-hour rhythm, reaching a peak in the middle of the usual sleep period (dark area). In physiological terms, the circadian factor is more likely to be a "wake drive" than a sleep drive (i.e., the inverse of the curve displayed), but the net effect on predicted sleep-wake balance would be the same. In entrained humans, the homeostatic and circadian sleep factors interact to ensure a single episode of consolidated sleep at night.
Source. Adapted from Borbely AA et al: "Processes Underlying the Regulation of the Sleep-wake Cycle," in *Circadian Clocks.* Edited by Takahashi J, Turek F, Moore R. New York, Kluwer Academic/Plenum, 2001, pp. 457–479.

tion of prior wakefulness. Sleep drive builds up during the course of the waking day and then decreases during subsequent sleep. Homeostatic sleep drive is proportional to the amount of delta EEG activity expressed during NREM sleep. The second regulatory factor, previously discussed, is the circadian rhythm. In humans, the circadian drive for sleep is highest toward the end of the usual sleep period, between the hours of approximately 5:00 A.M. and 9:00 A.M. (The circadian sleep drive may actually be better represented by a circadian drive for alertness, which is at a minimum during these times.) Homeostatic and circadian sleep factors typically function interactively. Homeostatic sleep drive builds up near the usual sleep time at night and ensures rapid entry into deep NREM sleep. As homeostatic sleep drive weakens during the middle of the night, circadian sleep drive increases, maintaining sleep for the second half of the sleep period.

Sleep and wakefulness are controlled by a number of widely distributed brain systems (Jones 2000; Pace-Schott and Hobson 2002). No single region of the brain is necessary or sufficient for the generation of sleep or wakefulness, and lesioned animals typically recover sleep or wake function within several weeks.

Brain regions critical for normal *wakefulness* include the histaminergic nuclei of the posterior hypothalamus, the cholinergic nuclei of the basal forebrain, and the noradrenergic and serotonergic nuclei of the ascending reticular activating system and the midbrain and pontine tegmentum. In addition, a recently discovered system promotes wakefulness through the activity of a peptide neurotransmitter called hypocretin or orexin (see Chapter 4, "Narcolepsy and Syndromes of Central Nervous System–Mediated Sleepiness"). The hypocretin system acts as a master regulator of wakefulness through its connections to cholinergic, aminergic, and histaminergic brain systems.

Regions critical for the generation of *NREM sleep* include a variety of ascending brainstem centers, including the solitary tract, that have both ventral projections through the basal forebrain and dorsal projections through the thalamus to the rest of the cortex. Corticothalamic circuits become hyperpolarized during NREM sleep and establish many of the EEG rhythms by which NREM sleep is identified. More recent research has focused on the ventrolateral preoptic area of the hypothalamus, which acts as a "sleep switch" through reciprocal interactions with wake-promoting centers described above (Saper et al. 2001). In addition, homeostatic sleep regulation may involve activity of extracellular adenosine in the basal forebrain.

Finally, *REM sleep* results from reciprocal interactions between brain stem cholinergic "REM on" nuclei and noradrenergic/serotonergic "REM off" nuclei in the pontine tegmentum.

Although a wide variety of neurotransmitters are involved in sleep-wake states, their activities are complicated and often apparently contradictory (Zoltoski et al. 1999). In general, neurotransmitters including acetylcholine, histamine, serotonin, norepinephrine, and hypocretin appear to promote wakefulness. On the other hand, γ-aminobutyric acid (GABA) and galanin are more strongly associated with inhibitory influences that promote NREM sleep. Other substances, including cytokines, prostaglandins, and various hormones also influence sleep-wake states.

Clinical Assessment of Sleep and Circadian Rhythm Disorders

History

The proper diagnosis and management of sleep complaints rests on an accurate clinical history. As with any other medical or psychiatric disorder, important elements of the history include the nature, severity, and frequency of the symptoms, duration of the complaint, associated impairments, and exacerbating and alleviating factors. However, sleep and circadian rhythm disorders also differ in some important ways from other clinical conditions. Aspects of the clinical history more specific to sleep and circadian rhythm disorders include the following:

- *24-hour history.* Because sleep and wakefulness affect each other, it is important to assess both nighttime and daytime symptoms in patients with sleep complaints. Evaluating the circumstances and contingencies of sleep is very important. For instance, it is important to examine activities that occur just before the individual usually goes to bed, which may point out sleep-incompatible behaviors. Sleep latency (the time it takes to fall asleep); the number, duration, and timing of midnight awakenings; and the presence of specific sleep symptoms, such as snoring, movements during sleep, and abnormal behaviors should all be assessed. The timing of awakening in the morning, the use of alarm clocks or other behavioral measures to wake up, and the amount of time it takes to fully awaken are also important. Daytime activities, including school, work, exercise, and home activities, should then be evaluated. The presence of daytime sleepiness, as indicated by struggling to stay awake, the presence of inadvertent sleep episodes, or the presence of daytime naps, should also be assessed on a routine basis.

- *Regularity and timing of sleep-wake behaviors over time.* Sleep symptoms may vary considerably from day to day. This variability may be important in diagnosis and treatment planning. In the case of circadian rhythm sleep disorders, abnormal timing of sleep is the defining symptom.
- *Bed partner history.* The sleep history should also include a report from the bed partner if one is present. Certain symptoms, including snoring and sleep behaviors, may not be evident to the person with the disorder itself.

Questionnaires

A variety of sleep history questionnaires may help to speed the clinical history. The Epworth Sleepiness Scale (ESS; Johns 1991) is one of the most widely used questionnaires in sleep medicine. It assesses the likelihood of falling asleep in specific behavioral situations and has a range of 0 (no sleepiness) to 24 (extreme sleepiness). The Pittsburgh Sleep Quality Index (PSQI; Buysse et al. 1989) is an 18-item self-rated scale that assesses overall sleep quality, with scores ranging from 0 (good sleep quality) to 21 (poor sleep quality). A score of >5 is often used to identify clinically significant sleep complaints. Even more important, *sleep-wake diaries* may give a more complete picture of the individual's sleep patterns and variability from day to day. Not infrequently, maintaining a sleep diary can help the individual identify patterns that may be contributing to sleep problems. Examples of two types of sleep-wake diaries are shown in Figure 1–4.

A. Graphic sleep diary

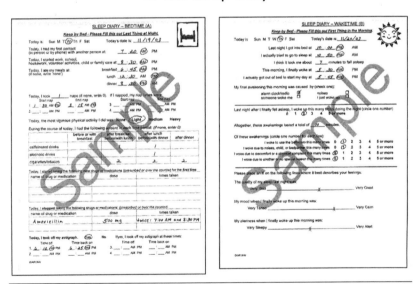

B. Text sleep diary

Figure 1–4. Sleep-wake diaries.

A: In a graphic sleep diary, the subject "blocks out" the times he or she was actually asleep. In this example, the subject had very irregular sleep timing with some very long sleep episodes. **B:** In a text sleep diary, the subject writes in the times of going to bed, waking up, napping, and so forth.

Actigraphy

Actigraphy refers to the measurement of body movements, typically through a wrist-worn activity meter. The pattern of motor activity corresponds reasonably well to sleep and wakefulness, although they are not identical. A number of studies have shown strong correlations between actigraphy and both sleep diaries and PSG, although actigraphy tends to overestimate sleep in comparison to PSG (Sadeh and Acebo 2002). The reason is that actigraphy cannot distinguish between an individual lying quietly awake and one who is actually asleep. An example of actigraphy output is shown in Figure 1–5.

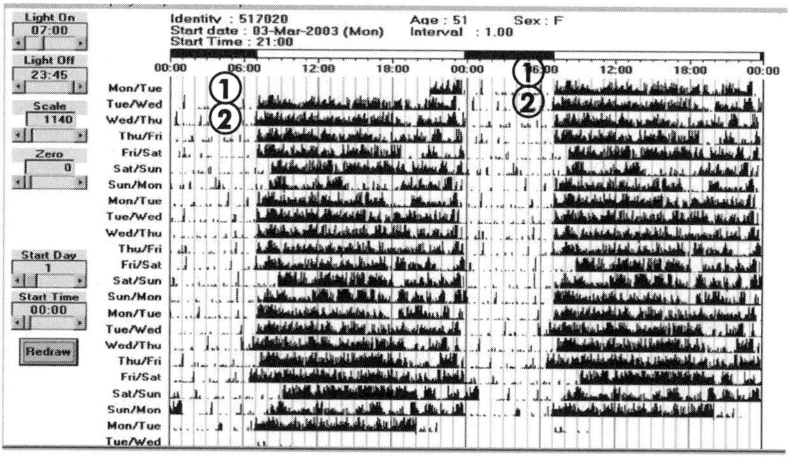

Figure 1–5.   Actigraphy data.

Actigraphy measures physical activity via a wrist-worn, motion-sensitive monitor. The output from an actigraph displays body movements as black peaks, and inactivity appears as a relatively blank area. By convention, data for each day are displayed twice, once to the right of, and once below the previous day. Activity for Day 1 and Day 2 are labeled to demonstrate this "double plotting," which facilitates the identification of patterns across days. In this example, the individual had a fairly regular rest-activity pattern, with inactivity (correlated with sleep) beginning at about midnight (00:00), and activity (correlated with wakefulness) beginning at about 7:00–8:00 A.M. (07:00–08:00). Period of low activity during the day may represent low-activity wakefulness or naps. Software can distinguish with sensitivity between these two possibilities.

Polysomnography

In addition to EEG, EOG, and EMG measurements, clinical poly-somnography typically includes a variety of other measures. These may include additional EEG channels; measurements of nasal-oral airflow or nasal pressure, together with measures of chest and abdominal movement to measure breathing and breathing pauses (apneas) during sleep; oximetry to measure de-saturation events accompanying sleep-disordered breathing; and additional EMG channels on the anterior tibialis muscles to as-sess for the presence of periodic limb movements during sleep, movements before sleep onset that characterize patients with restless legs syndrome, and parasomnias such as REM sleep be-havior disorder. An example of the channels in a clinical poly-somnogram is shown in Figure 1–6.

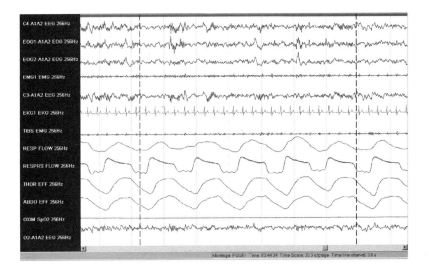

Figure 1–6.   Clinical polysomnogram.

A 30-second epoch of a typical clinical polysomnogram. In addition to electro-encephalographic (EEG; C4-A1A2, C3-A1A2, O2-A1A2), electrooculographic (EOG1-A1A2, EOG2-A1A2), and electromyographic (EMG1) recordings, a clin-ical polysomnogram includes additional channels for monitoring leg move-ments (anterior tibialis leads [TIBS EMG]), breathing patterns (nasal pressure [RESPRS], oral-nasal thermistors [RESP]), chest and abdominal wall move-ments (THOR EFF, ABDO EFF), oximetry (OXIM), and electrocardiogram (EKG1).

Polysomnography is indicated for the evaluation of patients with suspected sleep apnea. It may also be useful to evaluate patients with parasomnias, particularly when there is diagnostic uncertainty regarding the type of disorder. PSG is not routinely indicated for the assessment of insomnia, circadian rhythm sleep disorders, or restless legs syndrome. These disorders are typically based on clinical history, and PSG is reserved only for atypical or treatment-resistant cases (Chesson et al. 1997; Polysomnography Task Force 1997). Objective daytime sleepiness is assessed with a variant of PSG called the multiple sleep latency test (MSLT). A simplified polysomnographic montage (EEG, EOG, and EMG recordings) is used, and the patient is permitted to nap 4–5 times at 2-hour intervals during the day. The latency to sleep and the presence or absence of REM sleep are noted for each nap. The mean sleep latency serves as an overall measure of daytime sleepiness. Values >10 minutes are generally considered normal, values <8 minutes indicate clinically significant sleepiness, and values ≤5 indicate severe sleepiness. The presence of REM sleep in two or more naps suggests the possibility of narcolepsy (see Chapter 7, "Circadian Rhythm Sleep Disorders"). Prior sleep history (especially sleep deprivation), medications, and medication withdrawal can all affect MSLT results.

Disorders of Sleep and Wakefulness

Patients can typically present with one of four broad types of sleep-wake complaints: insomnia (complaint of difficulty falling or staying asleep), hypersomnia (complaint of excessive daytime sleepiness), parasomnias (abnormal behavioral or physiological events occurring during sleep), and circadian rhythm sleep disorders (disorders in the timing of sleep). Classification systems for sleep disorders include the *Diagnostic and Statistical Manual of Mental Disorders,* 4th Edition, Text Revision (DSM-IV-TR; American Psychiatric Association 2000), the *International Classification of Sleep Disorders* (ICSD; American Sleep Disorders Association 1997), and the *International Statistical Classification of Diseases and Related Health Problems,* 10th Revision (ICD-10; World Health Organization 1992). The ICD system groups sleep disorders into those of organic origin and those of mental origin. DSM-IV-TR classifies sleep disorders as primary or secondary. The ICSD describes categories of dyssomnias (which include insomnia, hypersomnia, and circadian rhythm sleep disorders), parasomnias, and secondary sleep disorders. A revised edition of the ICSD classifications (ICSD-2) is scheduled to be released in 2005 (American Academy of Sleep Medicine, personal communication, November 2004). In the ICSD-2, sleep disorders are categorized into one of six groups: insomnias, sleep-related breathing disorders, hypersomnias not due to a sleep-related breathing disorder, circadian rhythm sleep disorders, parasomnias, and sleep-related movement disorders.

The sleep disorders classified by any of these systems involve disorders presumed to be of neurologic, medical, and psychiatric or behavioral origins. Outlines of the DSM-IV-TR classification and the proposed ICSD-2 classification are provided in Table 1–2 and Table 1-3, respectively.

Overview of This Volume

The chapters in this volume are organized according to the major categories of sleep disorders that are likely to be encountered in psychiatric clinical practice: Chapter 2, "Insomnia" (Buysse and colleagues); Chapter 3, "Sleep Apnea" (Strollo and Davé); Chapter 4, "Narcolepsy and Syndromes of Central Nervous System–Mediated Sleepiness" (Black, Nishino, and Brooks); Chapter 5, "Restless Legs Syndrome" (Winkelman); Chapter 6, "Parasomnias" (Winkelman); and Chapter 7, "Circadian Rhythm Sleep Disorders" (Zee and Manthena). In each chapter, the authors discuss definitions and clinical description, epidemiology, etiology and pathogenesis, and treatment. Each chapter specifically addresses information of particular relevance to psychiatric clinicians. More detailed information on each of these disorders is available in general textbooks on sleep medicine (Chokroverty 1999; Kryger et al. 2000).

The field of sleep disorders medicine is broad and growing. One of the most exciting features of this field is that it provides psychiatric clinicians an opportunity to interact with specialists

Table 1–2. DSM-IV-TR sleep disorder classifications

Primary sleep disorders
Dyssomnias
 Primary insomnia
 Primary hypersomnia
 Narcolepsy
 Breathing-related sleep disorder
 Circadian rhythm sleep disorder (specify: delayed sleep phase
  type/jet lag type/shift work type/unspecified type)
 Dyssomnia NOS
Parasomnias
 Nightmare disorder
 Sleep terror disorder
 Sleepwalking disorder
 Parasomnia NOS
Sleep disorders related to another mental disorder
 Insomnia related to… *[indicate the Axis I or Axis II disorder]*
 Hypersomnia related to… *[indicate the Axis I or Axis II disorder]*
Other sleep disorders
 Sleep disorder due to… *[indicate the general medical condition]*
  Insomnia type
  Hypersomnia type
  Parasomnia type
  Mixed type
 Substance-induced sleep disorder *(use substance-specific codes)*

Note. NOS=not otherwise specified.
Source. Reprinted from American Psychiatric Association: *Diagnostic and Statistical Manual of Mental Disorders,* 4th Edition, Text Revision. Washington, DC, American Psychiatric Association, 2000. Used with permission.

from other areas of clinical medicine, including psychologists, pulmonologists, neurologists, and surgeons. Psychiatrists can frequently make important contributions to the care of patients with sleep disorders, given the importance of behavioral and psychopharmacologic interventions in managing these conditions. I hope this volume will provide practicing psychiatrists with the tools necessary to embark on these fruitful collaborations.

Table 1–3. Proposed International Classification of Sleep Disorders, 2nd Edition (ICSD-2)

I. **Insomnias**

   1. Adjustment insomnia (acute insomnia)

   2. Psychophysiological insomnia

   3. Paradoxical insomnia

   4. Idiopathic insomnia

   5. Insomnia due to mental disorder

   6. Inadequate sleep hygiene

   7. Behavioral insomnia of childhood

   8. Insomnia due to drug or substance

   9. Insomnia due to medical condition

  10. Insomnia not due to substance or known physiological condition, unspecified (nonorganic insomnia, NOS)

  11. Physiological (organic) insomnia, unspecified

II. **Sleep-related breathing disorders**

Central sleep apnea syndromes

   1. Primary central sleep apnea

   2. Central sleep apnea due to Cheyne Stokes breathing pattern

   3. Central sleep apnea due to high-altitude periodic breathing

   4. Central sleep apnea due to medical condition not Cheyne Stokes

   5. Central sleep apnea due to drug or substance

   6. Primary sleep apnea of infancy (formerly primary sleep apnea of newborn)

Obstructive sleep apnea syndromes

   7. Obstructive sleep apnea, adult

   8. Obstructive sleep apnea, pediatric

Sleep-related hypoventilation/hypoxemic syndromes

   9. Sleep-related nonobstructive alveolar hypoventilation, idiopathic

  10. Congenital central alveolar hypoventilation syndrome

Table 1–3. Proposed International Classification of Sleep Disorders, 2nd Edition (ICSD-2) *(continued)*

II. Sleep-related breathing disorders *(continued)*

Sleep-related hypoventilation/hypoxemia due to medical condition

11. Sleep-related hypoventilation/hypoxemia due to pulmonary parenchymal or vascular pathology

12. Sleep-related hypoventilation/hypoxemia due to lower airways obstruction

13. Sleep-related hypoventilation/hypoxemia due to neuromuscular and chest wall disorders

Other sleep-related breathing disorder

14. Sleep apnea/sleep-related breathing disorder, unspecified

III. Hypersomnias of central origin not due to a circadian rhythm sleep disorder, sleep-related breathing disorder, or other cause of disturbed nocturnal sleep

1. Narcolepsy with cataplexy

2. Narcolepsy without cataplexy

3. Narcolepsy due to medical condition

4. Narcolepsy, unspecified

5. Recurrent hypersomnia

   a. Kleine-Levin syndrome

   b. Menstrual-related hypersomnia

6. Idiopathic hypersomnia with long sleep time

7. Idiopathic hypersomnia without long sleep time

8. Behaviorally induced insufficient sleep syndrome

9. Hypersomnia due to medical condition

10. Hypersomnia due to drug or substance

11. Hypersomnia not due to substance or known physiological condition (nonorganic hypersomnia, NOS)

12. Physiological (organic) hypersomnia, unspecified origin (organic hypersomnia, NOS)

Table 1–3. Proposed International Classification of Sleep Disorders, 2nd Edition (ICSD-2) *(continued)*

IV. **Circadian rhythm sleep disorders**

  1. Circadian rhythm sleep disorder, delayed sleep phase type (delayed sleep phase disorder)
  2. Circadian rhythm sleep disorder, advanced sleep phase type (advanced sleep phase disorder)
  3. Circadian rhythm sleep disorder, irregular sleep-wake type (irregular sleep-wake rhythm)
  4. Circadian rhythm sleep disorder, nonentrained type (free-running or non–24-hour sleep-wake rhythm)
  5. Circadian rhythm sleep disorder, jet lag type (jet lag disorder)
  6. Circadian rhythm sleep disorder, shift work type (shift work disorder)
  7. Circadian rhythm sleep disorders due to medical condition
  8. Other circadian rhythm sleep disorder (circadian rhythm sleep disorder, NOS)
  9. Other circadian rhythm sleep disorder due to drug or substance

V. **Parasomnias**

  Disorders of arousal (from non-REM sleep)

  1. Confusional arousals
  2. Sleepwalking
  3. Sleep terrors

  Parasomnias usually associated with REM sleep

  4. REM sleep behavior disorder (including parasomnia overlap disorder and status dissociatus)
  5. Recurrent isolated sleep paralysis
  6. Nightmare disorder

  Other parasomnias

  7. Sleep-related dissociative disorders
  8. Sleep enuresis
  9. Sleep-related groaning (catathrenia)
  10. Exploding head syndrome
  11. Sleep-related hallucinations

Table 1–3. Proposed International Classification of Sleep Disorders, 2nd Edition (ICSD-2) *(continued)*

V. Parasomnias *(continued)*

Other parasomnias (continued)

12. Sleep-related eating disorder
13. Parasomnia, unspecified
14. Parasomnias due to drug or substance
15. Parasomnias due to medical condition

VI. Sleep-related movement disorders

1. Restless legs syndrome
2. Periodic limb movement disorder
3. Sleep-related leg cramps
4. Sleep-related bruxism
5. Sleep-related rhythmic movement disorder
6. Sleep-related movement disorder, unspecified
7. Sleep-related movement disorder due to drug or substance
8. Sleep-related movement disorder due to medical condition

VII. Isolated symptoms, apparently normal variants, and unresolved issues

1. Long sleeper
2. Short sleeper
3. Snoring
4. Sleep talking
5. Sleep starts (hypnic jerks)
6. Benign sleep myoclonus of infancy
7. Hypnagogic foot tremor and altenating leg muscle activation during sleep
8. Propriospinal myoclonus at sleep onset
9. Excessive fragmentary myoclonus

Note. REM=rapid eye movement.
Source. American Academy of Sleep Medicine, personal communication, November 2004.

References

American Psychiatric Association: Diagnostic and Statistical Manual of Mental Disorders, 4th Edition, Text Revision. Washington, DC, American Psychiatric Association, 2000

American Sleep Disorders Association: International Classification of Sleep Disorders, Revised: Diagnostic and Coding Manual. Rochester, MN, American Sleep Disorders Association, 1997

Belenky G, Wesensten NJ, Thorne DR, et al: Patterns of performance degradation and restoration during sleep restriction and subsequent recovery: a sleep dose-response study. J Sleep Res 12:1–12, 2003

Buysse DJ, Reynolds CF, Monk TH, et al: The Pittsburgh Sleep Quality Index (PSQI): a new instrument for psychiatric research and practice. Psychiatry Res 28:193–213, 1989

Carskadon MA, Dement WC: Normal human sleep: an overview, in Principles and Practice of Sleep Medicine, 3rd Edition. Edited by Kryger MH, Roth T, Dement WC. Philadelphia, PA, WB Saunders, 2000, pp 15–25

Chesson AL Jr, Ferber RA, Fry JM, et al: The indications for polysomnography and related procedures. Sleep 20:423–487, 1997

Chokroverty S (ed): Sleep Disorders Medicine: Basic Science, Technical Considerations, and Clinical Aspects, 2nd Edition. Boston, MA, Butterworth-Heinemann, 1999

Czeisler CA, Khalsa SB: The human circadian timing system and sleep-wake regulation, in Principles and Practice of Sleep Medicine, 3rd Edition. Edited by Kryger MH, Roth T, Dement WC. Philadelphia, PA, WB Saunders, 2000, pp 353–376

Czeisler CA, Duffy JF, Shanahan TL, et al: Stability, precision, and near-24-hr period of the human circadian pacemaker. Science 284:2177–2181, 1999

DeCoursey PJ, Walker JK, Smith SA: A circadian pacemaker in free-living chipmunks: essential for survival? J Comp Physiol [A] 186:169–180, 2000

Harrison Y, Horne JA: The impact of sleep deprivation on decision making: a review. J Exp Psychol Appl 6:236–249, 2000

Johns MW: A new method for measuring daytime sleepiness: the Epworth Sleepiness Scale. Sleep 14:540–545, 1991

Jones BE: Basic mechanisms of sleep-wake states, in Principles and Practice of Sleep Medicine, 3rd Edition. Edited by Kryger MH, Roth T, Dement WC. Philadelphia, PA, WB Saunders, 2000, pp 134–154

King DP, Takahashi JS: Molecular genetics of circadian rhythms in mammals. Annu Rev Neurosci 23:713–742, 2000

Kripke DF, Garfinkel L, Wingard DL, et al: Mortality associated with sleep duration and insomnia. Arch Gen Psychiatry 59:131–136, 2002

Kryger MH, Roth T, Dement WC (eds): Principles and Practice of Sleep Medicine, 3rd Edition. Philadelphia, PA, WB Saunders, 2000

Nofzinger EA, Mintun MA, Wiseman M, et al: Forebrain activation in REM sleep: an FDG PET study. Brain Res 770:192–201, 1997

Pace-Schott EF, Hobson JA: The neurobiology of sleep: genetics, cellular physiology and subcortical networks. Nat Rev Neurosci 3:591–605, 2002

Peppard PE, Young T, Palta M: Prospective study of the association between sleep-disordered breathing and hypertension. N Engl J Med 342:1378–1384, 2000

Pilcher JJ, Huffcutt AI: Effects of sleep deprivation on performance: a meta-analysis. Sleep 19:318–326, 1996

Polysomnography Task Force, American Sleep Disorders Association Standards of Practice Committee: Practice parameters for the indications for polysomnography and related procedures. Sleep 20:406–422, 1997b

Rechtschaffen A, Bergmann BM, Everson CE, et al: Sleep deprivation in the rat, X: integration and discussion of findings. Sleep 25:68–87, 1989

Riemann D, Voderholzer U: Primary insomnia: a risk factor to develop depression? J Affect Disord 76:255–259, 2003

Sadeh A, Acebo C: The role of actigraphy in sleep medicine. Sleep Med Rev 6:113–124, 2002

Saper CB, Chou TC, Scammell TE: The sleep switch: hypothalamic control of sleep and wakefulness. Trends Neurosci 24:726–731, 2001

Spiegel K, Leproult R, Van Cauter E: Impact of sleep debt on metabolic and endocrine function. Lancet 354:1435–1439, 1999

Spiegel K, Sheridan JF, Van Cauter E: Effect of sleep deprivation on response to immunization. JAMA 12:1471–1472, 2002

Stickgold R, Whidbee D, Schirmer B, et al: Visual discrimination task improvement: a multi-step process occurring during sleep. J Cogn Neurosci 12:246–254, 2000

Turner RS: Idiopathic rapid eye movement sleep behavior disorder is a harbinger of dementia with Lewy bodies. J Geriatr Psychiatry Neurol 15:195–199, 2002

VanDongen HP, Maislin G, Mullington JM, et al: The cumulative cost of additional wakefulness: dose-response effects on neurobehavioral functions and sleep physiology from chronic sleep restriction and total sleep deprivation. Sleep 26:117–126 [erratum, 27:600], 2003

World Health Organization: International Statistical Classification of Diseases and Related Health Problems, 10th Revision. Geneva, World Health Organization, 1992

Zoltoski RK, de Jesus Cabeza R, Gillin JC: Biochemical pharmacology of sleep, in Sleep Disorders Medicine: Basic Science, Technical Considerations, and Clinical Aspects, 2nd Edition. Edited by Chokroverty S. Boston, MA, Butterworth-Heinemann, 1999, pp 63–94

Chapter 2

Insomnia

Daniel J. Buysse, M.D.
Anne Germain, Ph.D.
Douglas Moul, M.D.
Eric A. Nofzinger, M.D.

Insomnia is one of the most prevalent health complaints in the general population, in medical practice, and in psychiatric practice. For many years, clinicians have been encouraged to think of insomnia as a symptom rather than a disorder, hoping to treat insomnia by finding and treating the underlying "cause."

Recent evidence has called this practice into question. Although insomnia is very commonly associated with other psychiatric and mental disorders, its onset, response to treatment, and long-term course are often independent of comorbid conditions. Furthermore, insomnia is independently associated with substantial morbidity, functional impairment, and health care costs. Finally, psychological, behavioral, and pharmacologic treatments for "primary" insomnia are also efficacious in "secondary" insomnias, potentially improving the comorbid conditions as well. Therefore, insomnia is increasingly viewed not simply as a symptom, but as a syndrome or disorder that frequently co-occurs with other medical and psychiatric conditions and that merits independent treatment.

Work on this chapter was supported by National Institutes of Health grants AG00972, AG29677, MH24652, MH61566, MH66227, and RR00052.

Definitions

Insomnia symptoms refer to complaints of difficulty falling asleep, frequent or prolonged awakenings, inadequate sleep quality, or short overall sleep duration in an individual who has adequate time available for sleep. Insomnia is not defined by sleep laboratory measures or a specific sleep duration. Because insomnia occurs only when there is adequate opportunity for sleep, it should be distinguished from *sleep deprivation,* in which the individual has relatively normal sleep ability but has inadequate opportunity for sleep.

An *insomnia disorder* is a syndrome consisting of the insomnia complaint together with significant impairment or distress and the exclusion of other causes. The most common daytime impairments associated with insomnia include complaints of mood disturbances, impaired cognitive function, and daytime fatigue (Moul et al. 2002). Typical mood symptoms are irritability, mild dysphoria, and difficulty tolerating stress. Cognitive complaints include difficulties in concentrating, completing tasks, and performing complex, abstract, or creative tasks. Fatigue is a common complaint in individuals with insomnia disorders, but actual daytime sleepiness is less common. In fact, many individuals with insomnia are unable to sleep during the day even though they feel tired.

Epidemiology and Consequences

The epidemiology of insomnia is complicated by several factors, including the distinction of symptom from disorder. First, because epidemiologic studies of sleep disorders rely on self-reports, biases may occur because of inexact wording of questions, length or form of interview, subjects' avoidance or exaggeration of symptoms, measurement of confounding comorbidities, concurrent medication use, and memory difficulties (Moul et al. 2004). In addition, deciding when a complaint is clinically significant is a challenge for epidemiological and clinical studies. Finally, the validity of epidemiological estimates of specific insomnia disorders may be limited by the low degree of interrater reliability of clinical diagnoses (Buysse et al. 1994). In-depth reviews of insomnia epidemiology are available elsewhere (Ohayon 2002), but major findings are reviewed below.

The one-year prevalence of insomnia symptoms in the United States and other Western nations is approximately 30%–40% in the general population and up to 66% in primary care and psychiatric settings. The prevalence of primary insomnia as a specific disorder is in the range of 5%–10% of the general population. Aside from estimating the prevalence of nighttime symptoms or syndromal insomnias, investigators continue to expand the study of daytime symptoms in primary insomnia, among them poor concentration, fatigue, dysphoria, sleep dissatisfaction, and mental inefficiency (Moul et al. 2002).

Risk factors for insomnia can be categorized into predisposing, initiating, and maintaining factors (Spielman et al. 1987). Established vulnerability factors include advancing age, female sex, being divorced or separated, unemployment, and comorbid medical and psychiatric illness. Genetic factors, although inadequately studied, represent another possible risk. Factors that commonly initiate or maintain insomnia include psychosocial stresses such as moves, relationship difficulties, occupational and financial problems, and caregiving responsibilities (Kappler and Hohagen 2003). An additional maintaining factor that forms the basis for many therapeutic interventions is the adoption of counterproductive sleep habits (described later in this chapter). It remains difficult to estimate the exact roles of different risk factors in the initiation and maintenance of insomnia in specific populations.

The natural history of insomnia, determined from population-based studies, has not been well described. However, follow-up studies of clinical patients and population samples indicate that insomnia often persists for years and may become more severe with time (Mendelson 1995; Vollrath et al. 1989), although remission has been described in one study of older adults (Foley et al. 1999). The longitudinal epidemiology of insomnia is complicated by normal aging, which leads to lighter and more fragmented sleep. Studies of older adults again suggest that insomnia is strongly related to medical and psychiatric conditions and that it decreases when these problems are adequately treated (Katz and McHorney 1998).

The consequences of insomnia can be substantial. Several studies have identified insomnia as a risk factor for the later development of depressive, anxiety, and substance use disorders (Breslau et al. 1996; Chang et al. 1997; reviewed in Riemann and Voderholzer 2003). In patients with major depressive disorder (MDD), insomnia is associated with worse treatment outcomes (Buysse et al. 1999), suicidal ideation (Agargun et al. 1997), symptom persistence (Moos and Cronkite 1999), and recurrence of MDD (Perlis et al. 1997a; Reynolds et al. 1997). Insomnia is also associated with persistence and relapse in alcohol dependence (Brower et al. 2001). Insomnia is associated with increased medical care utilization, more absenteeism from work (Simon and Von Korff 1997), and increased direct and indirect medical costs (Walsh and Engelhardt 1999). Insomnia may be associated with increased motor vehicle and other accidents (Powell et al. 2002), as well as increased incidence of falls in the elderly (Brassington et al. 2000).Various studies have also substantiated reduced quality of life in individuals with insomnia (Hatoum et al. 1998; Léger et al. 2001) that is similar in magnitude to that seen with chronic conditions such as congestive heart failure and MDD (Katz and McHorney 2002). Quality of life is associated with the severity of the insomnia complaint, and in individuals with medical disorders, quality of life has an effect independent of the comorbid condition (Karlsen et al. 1999; McCall et al. 2000). Quality of life problems among individuals with insomnia include role impairments across a broad set of domains such as job performance, social life, and family life (Léger et al. 2002).

Pathophysiology and Etiology

Physiological Models

Insomnia is often considered to be a disorder of increased arousal. *Arousal* may refer to many different phenomena, but a working definition of arousal is the individual's state of central nervous system (CNS) activity and reactivity, ranging from sleep at one end of the spectrum to wakefulness with excitement or panic at the other (Coull 1998). Arousal is related to the function of wake-promoting structures in the ascending reticular activating system, hypothalamus, and basal forebrain, which interact with sleep-promoting brain centers in the anterior hypothalamus and thalamus (see Chapter 1, "Introduction"). *Hyperarousal* is a state characterized by a high level of alertness that may be present tonically or in response to specific situations, such as the sleep environment.

Psychophysiological and metabolic evidence for hyperarousal in insomnia patients includes findings of increased body temperature and galvanic skin response near sleep onset and increased heart rate and decreased heart period variability during sleep (reviewed in Bonnet and Arand 1997a). Whole-body metabolic rate measured by volume of oxygen consumption per unit of time (VO_2) is higher during sleep in patients with insomnia compared with healthy sleepers (Bonnet and Arand 1995, 1997b), again supporting the general concept of hyperarousal.

Electrophysiological evidence for hyperarousal comes from studies showing elevated high-frequency electroencephalographic (EEG) activity (beta activity) during non–rapid eye movement (NREM) sleep in insomnia patients (Krystal et al. 2002; Merica et al. 1998; Perlis et al. 2001). Beta activity is normally associated with mental activity during wakefulness. Reduced homeostatic sleep drive in insomnia patients, indicated by reduced delta EEG activity, has been found in some studies as well (Merica and Gaillard 1992).

Neuroendocrine evidence for hyperarousal includes increased cortisol and adrenocorticotropic hormone levels before and during sleep, particularly during the first half of sleep, in insomnia patients (Rodenbeck et al. 2002; Vgontzas et al. 2001). Decreased melatonin levels have been found less consistently (Attenburrow et al. 1996; Hajak et al. 1995).

Finally, hyperarousal is suggested by *functional neuroanatomic studies of arousal,* as indicated by patterns of regional brain metabolic activity during NREM sleep during single-photon emission computed tomography (SPECT) and positron emission tomography (PET) scans. In the first PET study of primary insomnia, patients had increased global glucose metabolic rates during both wakefulness and sleep compared with healthy control subjects, and the usual sleep-related decline in metabolism in brainstem arousal centers was attenuated (Nofzinger et al. 2004) (Figure 2–1, part A). During wakefulness, primary insomnia patients have reduced dorsolateral prefrontal cortical activity. This constellation of findings suggests hyperarousal during NREM sleep and frontal hypoarousal during wakefulness, which may correspond to patients' sleep- and wake-related complaints (Figure 2–1, part B). In patients with insomnia in the context of major depression, EEG beta activity was positively associated with metabolic activity in the orbitofrontal cortex and with complaints of poor sleep quality (Nofzinger et al. 2000), further substantiating the hyperarousal hypothesis. On the other hand, a study using [^{99m}Tc]-HMPAO SPECT in primary insomnia patients (M.T. Smith et al. 2002a) found hypoperfusion across eight preselected regions of interest (including frontal medial, occipital, and parietal cortex) during NREM sleep, with the most prominent effects in the basal ganglia. Thus, imaging studies have begun to show functional neuroanatomic changes during NREM sleep associated with primary and secondary insomnia, although the precise nature of these changes awaits further confirmation.

Cognitive-Behavioral Models

All cognitive-behavioral models of insomnia outline the relationships between sleep-related thoughts, behaviors, and perceived arousal, their antecedents, and their consequences. However, the core dysfunction underlying insomnia differs across models. In the behavioral model of Spielman et al. (1987) (Figure 2–2), individual predisposing factors (e.g., heightened physiological or cognitive arousal) interact with external precipitating factors (e.g., life stressors) to produce insomnia. Perpetuating factors (e.g., maladaptive coping strategies such as spending more time in bed) maintain and reinforce insomnia even after the original precipitants recede.

In Morin's (1993) model, cognitive hyperarousal, indicated by sleep-focused, ruminative thoughts, particularly around bedtime, is the central component. Cognitive arousal increases physiological arousal. With repetition, this pairing facilitates conditioning between temporal (e.g., bedtime routines) and envi-

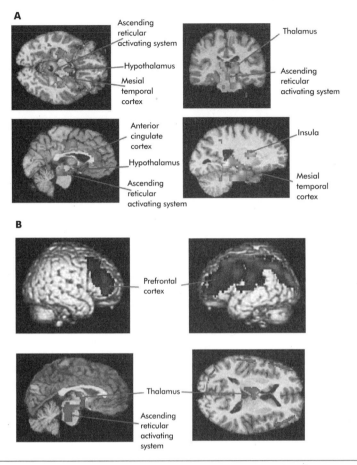

Figure 2–1. Positron emission tomography (PET) study of primary insomnia.

A: PET subtraction images comparing wakefulness and non–rapid eye movement (NREM) sleep in insomnia patients ($n=7$) and healthy control subjects ($n=20$). Relative glucose metabolism was measured in all subjects during wakefulness and again during NREM sleep. Relative glucose metabolism was lower during NREM sleep than during wakefulness in both groups. Dark brain regions indicate areas where insomnia patients had smaller wake–NREM differences compared with healthy control subjects. These results indicate that insomnia patients had less functional deactivation of alerting structures during NREM sleep. **B:** Brain structures where relative metabolism during wakefulness is lower in insomnia patients than in healthy subjects. These results suggest "hypoarousal" of cortical and brainstem structures during wakefulness, which may correspond to some of the daytime complaints of insomnia patients. Differences for all regions shown reach statistical significance at $P<0.05$, corrected.
Source. Adapted from Nofzinger et al. 2004.

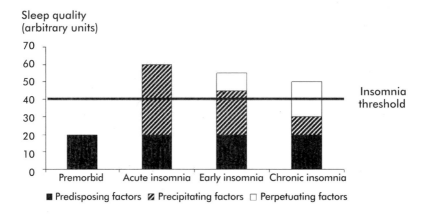

Figure 2–2. Heuristic model of the development of insomnia.

This behavioral model of insomnia proposes that individuals have varying predispositions for insomnia and that specific precipitating factors will lead vulnerable individuals to cross the insomnia threshold. Behavioral factors lead to perpetuation of the insomnia after the original precipitants have receded.

Source. Adapted from Spielman AJ: "Assessment of Insomnia." *Clinical Psychology Review* 6:11–25, 1986.

ronmental (e.g., bed, bedroom) cues and sleeplessness. Resulting sleep disturbance and ruminations ultimately lead to daytime consequences such as mood disturbances and fatigue. Over time, these experiences can alter one's beliefs regarding the ability to sleep and the consequences of sleep difficulties and can lead to the development of maladaptive strategies aimed at maximizing sleep (e.g., spending more time in bed) that further reinforce sleep disturbances and cognitive hyperarousal.

Perlis and colleagues (1997b) proposed a neurocognitive model of insomnia to explain discrepancies between objective polysomnographic findings and subjective reports of poor sleep quality and sleep misperception. Specifically, this model emphasizes brain cortical arousal as a central component and suggests that both physiological and cognitive arousal arise from increased cortical arousal at or around the sleep onset period, as measured by beta EEG activity. The authors posited that this arousal can be conditioned and that it further contributes to the insomnia experience.

Another cognitive model, by Harvey (2002), emphasizes the role of attention biases in the maintenance of insomnia. The model proposes that cognitive strategies (rather than behavioral strategies) employed by people with insomnia are maladaptive and maintain sleep disturbances. Excessive negative cognitive activity leads to increased physiological hyperarousal, which in turn leads to selective attention to and monitoring of autonomic symptoms and environmental cues indicative of sleeplessness. Such selective attention distorts perceptions regarding sleep deficits and adverse daytime effects. Individuals develop maladaptive safety behaviors, such as thought suppression and emotional inhibition, to avoid sleep loss. However, these behaviors further reinforce the negative cognitive activity, physiological arousal, and erroneous beliefs regarding sleep and daytime deficits seen in insomnia.

Clinical Assessment and Diagnosis

History

The assessment of patients with insomnia rests on a detailed clinical history. As with any clinical disorder, the history for insomnia should focus on specific symptoms, chronology, exacerbating and alleviating factors, and response to previous treatments. However, some aspects of the insomnia history differ from those of other disorders and deserve special emphasis.

1. The insomnia history should include a 24-hour perspective, covering the patient's usual sleep and wake periods. This history should include consideration of behaviors, cognitions, and environmental factors related to bedtime.
2. Regularity or variability of sleep hours from day to day should be established.
3. Symptoms of specific sleep disorders, such as restless legs syndrome, snoring or breathing problems during sleep, pain or limitations to mobility during sleep, and the presence of abnormal behaviors (parasomnias; see Chapter 6 in this volume) should be assessed.
4. Daytime activities should be reviewed, with particular emphasis on exercise routines, regularity of work and daytime activities, limitations in these activities, and daytime sleepiness and napping.

Table 2–1.   Medical and neurologic diseases associated with insomnia

Type of disease/disorder	Possible cause(s) for insomnia
Cardiovascular	
Congestive heart failure	Central sleep apnea, orthopnea
Coronary artery disease	Angina (may occur during sleep)
Pulmonary	
COPD	Breathing difficulty; sleep apnea
Asthma	Asthma attacks commonly occur during sleep
Neurologic	
Stroke	Damage to sleep-regulating brain structures; mobility limitations
Parkinson's disease	Mobility limitation; direct effects of impaired dopamine neurotransmission; periodic limb movement disorder
Neuropathy	Pain
Traumatic brain injury	Damage to sleep-regulating brain structures
Gastrointestinal	
Gastroesophageal reflux	Pain, initiation of apneas
Renal	
Chronic renal failure	Restless legs syndrome; obstructive sleep apnea
Endocrine	
Diabetes	Associated obesity, sleep apnea; neuropathy
Hyperthyroidism	Hyperarousal
Rheumatologic	
Rheumatoid arthritis, osteoarthritis	Pain, microarousals, high-frequency EEG activity during NREM sleep
Fibromyalgia	Pain, microarousals, high-frequency EEG activity during NREM sleep

Note.   COPD=chronic obstructive pulmonary disease; EEG= electroencephalographic; NREM=non–rapid eye movement.

Table 2–2. Common medications and substances associated with insomnia

Drug/substance	Comments
Alcohol	Intoxication associated with short sleep latency and increased slow-wave sleep in first half of night, but increased wakefulness and rapid eye movement (REM) in second half
	Alcohol dependence associated with insomnia, reduced slow-wave sleep
	Acute withdrawal associated with severe insomnia, REM sleep rebound
Caffeine	Patients with insomnia may be very sensitive to even small doses; contained not only in coffee and tea, but also in colas and other soft drinks, chocolate, and some aspirin products
Nicotine	Both use and withdrawal have been associated with insomnia
Antidepressants	Several classes may be associated with insomnia, including selective serotonin reuptake inhibitors, venlafaxine, bupropion, secondary tricyclics (desipramine)
Decongestants	Contain phenylephrine or pseudoephedrine
Corticosteroids	Insomnia typically associated with acute administration
β-Agonist and theophylline-derivative bronchodilators	Theophylline is a methylxanthine, like caffeine
β-Antagonists	Lipophilic compounds (e.g., propranolol) may cause insomnia and/or nightmares
Stimulants[a]	May cause insomnia in children and adults treated for attention-deficit/hyperactivity disorder
Statins	Few reports of insomnia, no polysomnographic data available

[a]Methylphenidate, dextroamphetamine, mixed amphetamine salts.

5. Interviewing the patient's bedpartner may be useful, because some aspects of sleep (such as periodic leg movements or parasomnias) may not be evident to the patient.
6. A thorough medical and psychiatric history is also important in the evaluation of insomnia. Medical conditions that cause breathing difficulty, pain, or limited mobility may be especially important in establishing an insomnia complaint. Table 2–1 lists common medical conditions associated with insomnia. Virtually any psychiatric disorder can also be associated with insomnia, but mood disorders, anxiety disorders, and psychotic disorders are most frequently comorbid with insomnia.
7. Finally, a thorough medication and substance history is essential and should include information about prescription and over-the-counter medications, substances such as caffeine and alcohol, and drugs of abuse. The list of medications that can be potentially associated with insomnia is long; it is summarized in Table 2–2.

Other Assessment Tools

Although the clinical history is the key to making an insomnia diagnosis, several other tools may aid this process.

Sleep-wake diaries covering 1 or 2 weeks, in which patients record their actual sleep hours and sleep experiences, can be invaluable. Diaries are useful for establishing patterns of sleep, as well as for indicating the day-to-day variability in sleep hours and sleep problems. An example of a sleep diary for insomnia patients is shown in Figure 1–4 in Chapter 1.

Actigraphy is an objective means of assessing rest-activity patterns by use of a motion-sensitive device worn on the nondominant wrist. Commercially available software provides descriptive statistics and graphical displays of rest-activity patterns. Validation studies have shown a strong correlation between actigraphy patterns and sleep as monitored by polysomnography (PSG), although actigraphy tends to overestimate the actual amount of sleep (Sadeh and Acebo 2002). Like the sleep diary, actigraphy can be useful for examining temporal patterns, variability, and responses to treatment.

Polysomnography, or a sleep study, is the gold standard for quantifying sleep and sleep disturbances. PSG is not routinely recommended for the evaluation of chronic insomnia (Sateia et al. 2000) because in most cases, PSG simply confirms the patient's subjective report without indicating a cause for awakenings. However, PSG may be useful in specific situations involving patients with symptoms of sleep apnea (see Chapter 3), periodic limb movements (Chapter 5), or parasomnias (Chapter 6). Patients who have atypical complaints or a history of poor response to usually efficacious treatments may be candidates for polysomnography.

Differential Diagnosis

Many classifications have been proposed for insomnia, some based on symptoms, others on duration, and still others on presumed etiology.

- *Symptom-based classifications* (i.e., sleep-onset, sleep maintenance, or mixed-type insomnia) are of limited value because the specific type of sleep complaint often varies within an individual over time (Hohagen et al. 1994a) and a majority of patients actually complain of more than one type of sleep disturbance.
- *Duration-based classifications* (e.g., acute, short-term, and chronic insomnia) are also of limited value because of the high rate of chronicity or recurrence in insomnia symptoms. Duration-based classification is most useful in that specific causes of insomnia may be associated with their duration. For instance, transient and short-term insomnias are often related to specific psychosocial or environmental stresses, whereas chronic insomnia is more often related to intrinsic sleep disorders or primary insomnia.
- *Etiology-based classifications* are the most useful for categorizing insomnia. Specific classification systems include the *International Statistical Classification of Diseases and Related Disorders,* 9th Revision (ICD-9) and 10th Revision (ICD-10; World Health Organization 1992), the *Diagnostic and Statistical Manual of*

Mental Disorders, 4th Edition, Text Revision (DSM-IV-TR; American Psychiatric Association 2000), and the *International Classification of Sleep Disorders,* Revised (ICSD; American Sleep Disorders Association 1997) and 2nd Edition (ICSD-2; American Academy of Sleep Disorders, in press).

In general, the ICD has the broadest, least well described categories, DSM-IV-TR has somewhat more specific categories, and ICSD has the most specific of all. However, each basically describes three major categories of insomnia:

1. *Insomnia secondary to other conditions.* This includes insomnias associated with medical disorders, insomnia related to mental disorders, and insomnia related to the acute effects of a substance or withdrawal from a substance/medication. This is the largest single group of chronic insomnia diagnoses seen in epidemiological studies and in clinical samples (Buysse et al. 1994; Ohayon 1997).
2. *Insomnia as a symptom of other specific sleep disorders.* This group includes the insomnia seen in restless legs syndrome, some cases of obstructive sleep apnea syndrome, and some cases of parasomnias. Insomnia, particularly difficulty in falling asleep, is a very frequent symptom of restless legs syndrome. Insomnia is somewhat less common in obstructive sleep apnea syndrome, although older adults and those with more central sleep apneas may have this presentation.
3. *Primary insomnia.* This category refers to disorders in which insomnia is the primary symptom and no other disorder is a possible cause. DSM-IV-TR includes a single category for primary insomnia. ICSD subdivides it into a number of categories, such as psychophysiological insomnia, idiopathic insomnia, and paradoxical insomnia.

Behavioral Treatment

Behavioral treatments aim to reduce sleep latency and improve sleep consolidation by changing behaviors and habits that interfere with sleep. A cognitive component is sometimes included to address distorted or maladaptive beliefs related to sleep. Behavioral treatments of insomnia can be administered in an individual or a group format.

Types of Treatments

Cognitive-behavioral interventions for insomnia are described in this section and are listed in Table 2–3.

Stimulus control therapy is based on principles of operant learning (Bootzin and Nicassio 1978) and aims to reinforce associations between sleepiness, sleep, and the sleep environment. The patient is instructed to use the bed and bedroom only for sleep and sex, and to go to the bedroom only when feeling sleepy. If awake for long periods of time in bed (e.g., 20 minutes or longer), the individual is instructed to get out of bed and leave the bedroom until feeling sleepy again.

Sleep restriction therapy involves restricting the time spent in bed by setting strict bedtime and rising schedules that closely match the number of hours of actual sleep reported by the patient (Spielman et al. 1987). The aim is to increase sleep efficiency, or the ratio of total time spent asleep to total time spent in bed. Initially, sleep restriction is often associated with slight to moderate sleep deprivation, which increases sleepiness and enhances the ability to fall asleep and to maintain sleep. Sleep restriction may lead to increased daytime sleepiness, and patients should be cautioned about operating machinery or performing duties that require high levels of alertness.

Relaxation techniques aim to reduce muscular tension and cognitive arousal, which are incompatible with sleep (Jacobson 1974; Woolfolk and McNulty 1983). Several specific relaxation techniques have been evaluated for insomnia. *Autogenic training* involves focusing on physiological sensations, such as heat, to induce relaxation via modulation of the autonomic nervous system. *Biofeedback* relies on a similar principle, but the process of reducing autonomic arousal is aided by the use of visual or auditory feedback to monitor biological signals such as heart rate or skin temperature to indicate arousal levels to the patient, who can then voluntarily reduce physiological arousal through active concentration. *Acupuncture* is distinct from conventional relax-

Table 2–3. Cognitive-behavioral interventions for insomnia

Intervention	General description	Specific techniques
Stimulus control	A set of behaviors that promotes associative conditioning between the sleep environment and sleepiness	• Go to bed only when feeling sleepy and intending to fall asleep. • If unable to fall asleep within 10–20 minutes (without watching the clock, 10–20 minutes is equivalent to repositioning yourself twice to try to fall asleep), leave the bed and the bedroom. Return only when feeling sleepy again. • Use the bed and bedroom for sleep only. Do not read, watch television, talk on the phone, worry, or plan activities in the bedroom. • Set the alarm and wake up at a regular time every day. • Do not snooze. Do not nap during the day.

Table 2-3. Cognitive-behavioral interventions for insomnia (*continued*)

Intervention	General description	Specific techniques
Sleep restriction therapy	Sleep practices that increase "sleep drive" and facilitate the ability to sleep	• Restrict time awake in bed by setting strict bedtime and rising schedules limited to the average number of hours of actual sleep reported in one night. • Increase time in bed by advancing bedtime by 15–30 minutes when the time spent asleep is at least 85% of the allowed time in bed. • Keep a fixed wakeup time, regardless of actual sleep duration. • If after 10 days sleep efficiency is lower than 85%, delay bedtime by 15–30 minutes.
Relaxation training	Training in techniques that decrease waking arousal and facilitate sleep at night. Muscular tension and cognitive arousal are incompatible with sleep.	• Practice muscle relaxation daily, using Jacobson's (1974) progressive relaxation training. • Use guided imagery to decrease rumination at bedtime by replacing arousing mental content and by deliberate avoidance of intrusive thoughts.

Table 2–3. Cognitive-behavioral interventions for insomnia (*continued*)

Intervention	General description	Specific techniques
Cognitive restructuring of irrational sleep-related beliefs	Identification, challenge, and replacement of dysfunctional beliefs and attitudes regarding sleep and sleep loss. These beliefs increase arousal and tension, which in turn impede sleep and reinforce the dysfunctional beliefs.	*Irrational beliefs and fears about sleep include* • Overestimation of number of hours of sleep one needs in order to be rested • Overall apprehensive expectation that sleep cannot be controlled • Fear of getting out of bed when awake for fear of missing the time when sleep will come
Sleep hygiene	Promotion of behaviors that improve sleep; limitation of behaviors that harm sleep	• Avoid naps. • Get regular exercise, at least 6 hours before sleep. • Maintain a regular sleep schedule 7 nights a week. • Avoid stimulants (caffeine, nicotine). • Limit alcohol intake. • Do not look at the clock when awake in bed.

ation and other behavioral techniques, but preliminary evidence suggests that it too may be efficacious for insomnia (see Sok et al. 2003 for meta-analysis).

Cognitive interventions involve the identification, challenge, and replacement of initial erroneous beliefs or fears regarding loss of sleep (Gross and Borkovec 1982). Cognitive distortions increase arousal and tension, further preventing sleep. Challenging the erroneous beliefs and fears can be done through education and discussion within a psychotherapeutic context. Replacing the irrational beliefs and fears requires behavioral changes to test the new beliefs and cognitive strategies to face resurgence of distorted thoughts about sleep. Cognitive therapy is most often combined with more behaviorally based interventions (Morin 1993). Paradoxical intention is another example of a cognitive technique used for insomnia. The rationale is that actively trying to maintain wakefulness will reduce performance anxiety related to falling asleep and thus will facilitate sleep onset. Data indicate that paradoxical intention may provide some benefit, but responses are highly variable (Morin et al. 1999).

Sleep hygiene refers to a set instructions aimed at reinforcing sleep-promoting behaviors and reducing the frequency of behaviors that may interfere with sleep (Hauri 1991). Exercising, relaxing evening routines, avoiding stimulants and naps, and limiting alcohol intake are examples of behaviors that may enhance sleep quality. Although sleep hygiene alone has limited efficacy to reduce insomnia (Lacks and Morin 1992), it is often combined with other behavioral interventions.

Efficacy of Behavioral Treatments

Behavioral interventions for insomnia significantly reduce sleep onset latency, reduce wake time after sleep onset, and improve total sleep time. Two meta-analyses support the efficacy of behavioral or cognitive-behavioral treatments of chronic insomnia (Morin et al. 1994; Murtagh and Greenwood 1995). Overall, a majority (70%–80%) of insomnia patients benefit from behavioral interventions, and improvements are maintained or enhanced at follow-up. Stimulus control, sleep restriction, and relaxation show the most robust effects among specific behavioral interventions. A third meta-analysis (Montgomery and Dennis 2003) investigated the efficacy of behavioral interventions in older adults. Overall, cognitive-behavioral therapy was effective at reducing sleep maintenance insomnia.

One additional meta-analysis (M.T. Smith et al. 2002b) compared the efficacy of cognitive-behavioral treatments and pharmacologic agents for insomnia. When compared with hypnotic medications, stimulus control and sleep restriction therapies were associated with similar improvements in wake time after sleep onset, number of awakenings, and sleep quality ratings. Behavioral interventions were associated with greater reductions in sleep onset latency, but hypnotics were associated with greater increases in total sleep time.

New Developments in Behavioral Treatments of Insomnia

New behavioral treatment modalities for insomnia are currently being investigated to disseminate these treatments and reduce patient burden and costs. These new developments include in-home visits (Espie et al. 2001), telephone interventions, Internet-based interventions (Strom et al. 2004), and self-help material (Mimeault and Morin 1999). Initial results suggest that behavioral interventions can be effectively delivered via these nontraditional methods. In elderly patients, however, one study suggest that in-person, group behavioral interventions may be more effective than home-based relaxation treatment to reduce insomnia complaints (Rybarczyk et al. 2002).

Psychological Treatment of Insomnia Secondary to Another Condition

Cognitive-behavioral interventions for insomnia are also effective at improving sleep quality in patients with comorbid medical and psychiatric illnesses (Lichstein et al. 2000) and specific conditions such as cancer (D'Ambrosio et al. 1999; Simeit et al. 2004) and chronic pain (Currie et al. 2000; Espie et al. 2001; Morin et al. 1989). Multifaceted psychological insomnia interventions have been shown to improve sleep quality in caregivers of dementia patients (McCurry and Ancoli-Israel 2003). A growing number of studies show that cognitive-behavioral treatments delivered in the primary and psychiatric care settings are also efficacious (Edinger and Sampson 2003; Espie et al. 2001).

Clinical Practice Points

Most of the behavioral treatments described above have been evaluated in clinical trials using approximately six 1-hour sessions delivered by trained therapists. However, these treatments share a few basic principles that can be used in a variety of clinical settings as a basic behavioral treatment package. These specific interventions are reasonable straightforward and rely on principles of the "two-process" model of sleep regulation (see Chapter 1, "Introduction") and simple conditioning. These recommendations are summarized in Table 2–4.

Pharmacologic Treatment

The only drugs currently approved for the treatment of insomnia are benzodiazepine receptor agonists (BzRA). However, physicians frequently use drugs from other classes to treat insomnia. Between the years 1987 and 1996, the use of antidepressants to treat insomnia increased by 146% and the use of BzRA fell by over 50% (Walsh and Schweitzer 1999). Data from the Verispan Physician Drug and Diagnosis Audit (Verispan, Yardley, PA) in 2002 showed an apparent continuation of this trend, with antidepressants accounting for 5.3 million prescriptions, compared with approximately 4.2 million for BzRA (Walsh 2004). However, the use of other medications for insomnia, such as antihistamines, antipsychotics, and anticonvulsants, is based on sparse efficacy and safety data.

Benzodiazepine Receptor Agonists

Indications

BzRA are indicated for the treatment of primary insomnia and its various subtypes, as well as for acute situational insomnia. They are useful as adjunctive therapies for secondary insomnia related

Table 2–4.   Brief behavioral treatment for insomnia

Behavioral intervention	Rationale
Limit time in bed to actual sleep time + 30 minutes (approximately).	Removing wakefulness from sleep period and lengthening duration of wakefulness increases homeostatic sleep drive.
Establish regular wake time every day, regardless of prior night's sleep duration.	Regular wake time promotes regular circadian sleep cycle, increases homeostatic sleep drive.
Do not go to bed until sleepy.	This technique increases homeostatic sleep drive, prevents frustration of lying awake in bed.
Do not stay in bed if awake for more than about 20 minutes.	This technique reduces frustration of lying awake in bed, prevents development of associations between bed and wakefulness.
Avoid caffeine and alcohol.	Both can disturb sleep.
Establish a physical exercise routine.	Aerobic exercise improves sleep depth, promotes regular daily schedule.

to certain medical conditions, psychiatric disorders, and other primary sleep disorders such as restless legs syndrome or circadian rhythm sleep disorders.

Pharmacodynamics

All BzRA bind at specific recognition sites on the γ-aminobutyric acid type A (GABA$_A$) receptor complex. GABA$_A$ receptors are widely distributed in the CNS, including in the cortex, basal ganglia, and cerebellum (Bateson 2004). GABA$_A$ receptors contain several components, including the GABA receptor itself, a benzodiazepine recognition site, and a chloride ion channel (Bateson 2004). The GABA receptor complex is made up of five protein subunits. These subunits belong to different families (alpha, beta, gamma, theta,

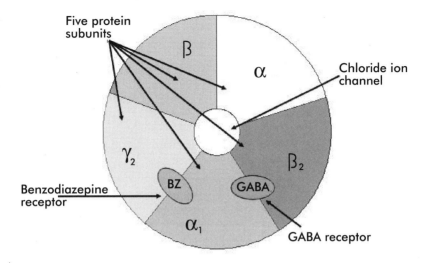

Figure 2–3. Benzodiazepine recognition site on the GABA receptor complex.

The γ-aminobutyric acid (GABA) receptor complex includes five protein subunits surrounding a chloride ion channel. Benzodiazepine receptor agonists bind at a specific recognition site at the interface of α and γ subunits. GABA itself binds at a different recognition site at the interface of α and β subunits.

epsilon, delta, pi, and rho), most of which also have two subtypes (e.g., α_{1-6}, β_{1-3}). Most $GABA_A$ receptors that are sensitive to BzRA include two alpha, two beta, and one gamma subunit. BzRA bind to a specific site at the interface of alpha and gamma subunits (Figure 2–3). Some BzRA, such as zolpidem and zaleplon, have relatively selective binding at $GABA_A$ receptors containing α_1 subunits. The clinical significance of this selectivity is not clear, although such agents may be relatively more specific for hypnotic effects and may have lower abuse liability. $GABA_A$ receptors with α_1 subunits are thought to mediate the sedative, amnestic, and anticonvulsant effects of BzRA, whereas those containing α_2 and α_3 subunits are more important for anxiolytic and myorelaxant effects (Mohler et al. 2002).

Pharmacokinetics

Although BzRA share a common mechanism of action, they have different clinical effects due to their different pharmacokinetic

Table 2–5. Benzodiazepine receptor agonists: pharmacokinetic properties

Drug	Onset of action (minutes)	Elimination half-life (hours)	Typical adult dose (mg)
Zaleplon	10–20	1.0	5–20
Zolpidem	10–20	1.5–2.4	5–10
Eszopiclone	10–30	5–6	1–3
Triazolam	10–20	1.5–5	0.125–0.25
Temazepam	45–60	8–20	7.5–30
Estazolam[a]	15–30	20–30	0.5–2
Quazepam[a]	15–30	15–120	7.5–15
Flurazepam[a]	15–30	36–120	15–30

[a]Has active metabolite.

properties for rate of absorption, extent of distribution, and terminal elimination half-life. These pharmacokinetic properties, together with dose, determine a drug's duration of action. Available agents range from those with half-lives of 1 hour (zaleplon) to those with half-lives of over 100 hours (flurazepam). Pharmacokinetic properties can be important in selecting a particular agent for a particular patient. For instance, a very short-acting drug such as zaleplon may be helpful for patients with predominantly sleep-onset problems, whereas longer-acting drugs such as temazepam may be more useful for nocturnal awakenings. Conversely, very short-acting drugs may wear off too soon, and longer-acting drugs may be associated with morning sedation. Table 2–5 shows the relevant clinical pharmacokinetic properties of BzRA commonly used to treat insomnia. Note that some of these drugs are not listed by the U.S. Food and Drug Administration as being indicated for insomnia but are still commonly used for this indication.

Effects on Sleep

BzRA share a common set of actions, including hypnotic, anxiolytic, myorelaxant, and anticonvulsant effects. BzRA decrease sleep latency, decrease the number and duration of awakenings during the middle of the night, and (for agents with longer duration of action) increase sleep duration (Parrino and Terzano 1996). Most BzRA slightly decrease the amount of Stage 3/4 NREM sleep, delta EEG activity, and REM sleep. Other effects include an increase in duration and frequency of sleep spindles during Stage 2 NREM sleep (see Chapter 1, "Introduction"). BzRA have inconsistent effects on the number of periodic limb movements during sleep, but they do reduce associated wakefulness (Saletu et al. 2001).

Efficacy

Several meta-analyses have demonstrated that the BzRA are efficacious in the treatment of chronic insomnia (Holbrook et al. 2000; Nowell et al. 1997; Soldatos et al. 1999) . On self-reported outcomes of sleep latency, sleep duration, number of awakenings, and sleep quality, BzRA are associated with effect sizes in the moderate to large range compared with placebo; this means that, on average, patients who are treated with BzRA in placebo-controlled trials show substantially more benefit than those treated with placebo. BzRA effects are comparable in magnitude to those of cognitive-behavioral therapies (M.T. Smith et al. 2002b).

A limitation of previous studies of BzRA has been their short overall duration. In the meta-analyses described above, the median duration of treatment was only 7 days. The brevity of these studies presents problems in terms of clinical utility, because the majority of patients treated with BzRA have chronic insomnia. One study demonstrated the efficacy of eszopiclone, compared with placebo, over 6 months of continued nightly use. The eszopiclone group had better outcomes in subjective sleep measures and in subjective daytime functioning (Krystal et al. 2003). This result suggests that BzRA may be efficacious over longer periods of time in at least some patients.

BzRA are often prescribed for intermittent use (e.g., to be used 3–5 times per week). Several studies have demonstrated the efficacy of zolpidem when used intermittently 3–5 times per week for up to 12 weeks (Perlis et al. 2004; Walsh et al. 2000a). Sleep outcomes for zolpidem pill nights were superior to outcomes for placebo pill nights and no-pill nights.

Side Effects

BzRA have common side effects, which differ somewhat depending on their pharmacokinetic properties. The major side effects of BzRA include the following:

- *Sedation.* This is the most common side effect of BzRA and is a result of the desired effect continuing into the desired wake period (Vermeeren 2004). Daytime sedation is related to duration of action, with longer-acting drugs causing more sedation.
- *Impaired psychomotor performance.* BzRA consistently impair motor speed and coordination, as judged by both laboratory test and simulated driving tasks. This impairment is most severe during the time that blood levels are high and is proportional to the duration, action, and half-life of the drug (Roehrs et al. 1994; Vermeeren 2004). Some studies have demonstrated an association between BzRA use and cognitive decline in older adults, but these findings are not consistent (Allard et al. 2003; Curran et al. 2003).
- *Falls and hip fractures.* BzRA have been consistently associated with falls and hip fracture in elderly persons (Cumming and Le Couteur 2003). However, many studies have not consistently accounted for the separate effect of insomnia, which has been found to be independently associated with falls and hip fractures (Brassington et al. 2000; Koski et al. 1998).
- *Motor vehicle accidents.* The bulk of evidence suggests increased risk of motor vehicle accidents among BzRA users (Thomas 1998), but findings have been somewhat inconsistent. Some studies have found only long-half-life BzRA to be associated with motor vehicle accidents, and others have found no association at all. Different indications (e.g., insomnia vs. anxiety) and administration patterns (e.g., once-daily nighttime use vs. multiple daytime doses) may also influence these results. As noted above, insomnia itself may also increase the risk of accidents (Powell et al. 2002).
- *Respiratory depression.* BzRA suppress respiration to a small degree, but this can become clinically significant in patients with severely impaired pulmonary function. Studies in patients with mild to moderate sleep apnea have shown little effect of

BzRA on oxyhemoglobin saturation or apnea-hypopnea index (Camacho and Morin 1995; Lofaso et al. 1997). (For a description of apnea-hypopnea index, see Chapter 3, "Sleep Apnea.")

The other side effects of BzRA—tolerance, discontinuance effects, and abuse—warrant special consideration.

- *Tolerance* has long been a concern with BzRA, but recent evidence calls into question whether this is an inevitable finding. Specifically, the 6-month study cited above (Krystal et al. 2003) showed no loss of efficacy over 6 months of continued nightly treatment, which is consistent with other data using self-report outcomes (Oswald et al. 1982) and with data from 5-week polysomnographic studies of zolpidem and zaleplon (Scharf et al. 1994; Walsh et al. 2000b). Similar findings have been observed with intermittent use of BzRA (Perlis et al. 2004; Walsh et al. 2000b). Epidemiologic studies show that up to two-thirds of patients taking hypnotics chronically report substantial ongoing benefit (Ohayon and Guilleminault 1999). Finally, a meta-analysis of BzRA effects showed an apparent loss of efficacy for triazolam, but not for zolpidem or zopiclone, after 2 weeks of continued nightly use, suggesting that the tolerance phenomenon may be more likely with some drugs than with others (Soldatos et al. 1999). In many placebo-controlled BzRA trials, placebo-treated groups show gradual improvements over time, which may account for some of the apparent loss of efficacy with BzRA treatment.
- *Discontinuance effects* are another potentially important side effect of BzRA. A number of studies have clearly shown rebound insomnia, defined as an increase in sleep problems to greater than the baseline level on discontinuation of the drug, but other studies have not. In the meta-analysis described above, triazolam and zolpidem were associated with rebound insomnia on the first night of discontinuation but not over the first 3 nights of discontinuation, suggesting that rebound insomnia is a short-lived phenomenon (Soldatos et al. 1999). Nevertheless, patients should be cautioned that abrupt discontinuation of these medications could lead to a worsening of symptoms that lasts for a few days.

- The potential for *abuse* is perhaps the greatest concern regarding benzodiazepines. Unfortunately, adequate and accurate data are not available to address this potential concern. Benzodiazepines have a marginal tendency for self-administration in animals, and this tendency is often used as a model of abuse potential in humans (Woods and Winger 1995). BzRA are rarely the drug of choice or sole drug of abuse in humans who abuse drugs. Nevertheless, individuals with a past history of substance abuse, particularly substance abuse of sedative-hypnotics or alcohol, remain at increased risk and should be treated cautiously with these medications (Griffiths and Weerts 1997).

Use of BzRA as Adjunctive Medications

Limited evidence suggests that BzRA are efficacious as adjunctive treatment in patients with comorbid medical and psychiatric disorders. For instance, zolpidem improved sleep time and wakefulness after sleep onset in depressed patients treated with selective serotonin reuptake inhibitors (Asnis et al. 1999), and clonazepam helped to reduce sleep symptoms without worsening the overall response in patients treated with fluoxetine (W. T. Smith et al. 2002).

Trazodone

Trazodone is a sedating antidepressant drug that is a weak but a specific inhibitor of the serotonin reuptake transporter, with minimal affinity for norepinephrine or dopamine reuptake. Trazodone also inhibits serotonin 5-HT_{1A}, 5-HT_{1C}, and 5-HT_2 receptors. Although it has no anticholinergic activity, it does have moderate antihistaminergic activity and is a weak antagonist of α_2 receptors and a somewhat more potent agonist of α_1 receptors (Golden et al. 2004). Trazodone is rapidly absorbed, with peak concentrations in 1–2 hours, and it has a half-life of approximately 5–9 hours. One of the metabolic products of trazodone is *m*-chlorophenylpiperazine (m-CPP), which itself possesses serotonergic activity and may be responsible for some of its side effects.

The sleep effects of trazodone have been described in small studies including control subjects and depressed patients, as well as one large study using only subjective outcomes in primary insomnia patients (reviewed in James and Mendelson 2004).

Sleep effects of trazodone and other nonbenzodiazepine medications used for insomnia are summarized in Table 2–6. Trazodone generally improves subjective sleep quality in healthy subjects and those with depression (Parrino et al. 1994; Saletu-Zyhlarz et al. 2002), but not consistently (van Bemmel et al. 1992). Trazodone has inconsistent effects in terms of improving PSG-defined sleep latency, wakefulness, total sleep time, and sleep efficiency (Saletu-Zyhlarz et al. 2002; van Bemmel et al. 1992). Unlike other sedating antidepressants, trazodone has little effect on REM sleep, with studies showing no significant change or a small decrease (Saletu-Zyhlarz et al. 2002; van Bemmel et al. 1992). Furthermore, trazodone is different from BzRA by virtue of increasing Stage 3/4 NREM sleep (Parrino et al. 1994; Saletu-Zyhlarz et al. 2002). In one large study comparing the effects of trazodone and zolpidem in patients with primary insomnia, trazodone improved subjective sleep latency, awakenings, wake time during sleep, and sleep time over 2 weeks of treatment, but these effects were significant only during the first week (Walsh et al. 1998).

Side effects of trazodone include sedation, orthostatic hypotension, lightheadedness, weakness, and the infrequent but serious risk of priapism.

Tricyclic Antidepressants

Sedating tricyclic antidepressants (TCAs) such as doxepin, trimipramine, and amitriptyline have been used in low doses to treat insomnia. Doxepin and amitriptyline inhibit both serotonin and norepinephrine reuptake transporters, but trimipramine has few such effects. Sedating TCAs also antagonize peripheral α_1- and α_2-adrenergic receptors. Finally, they are potent cholinergic and histamine antagonists. TCAs are rapidly absorbed, with maximum concentrations in 2–6 hours. Their half-lives range from 15 to 30 hours (Nelson 2004).

Table 2–6. Summary of nonbenzodiazepine drugs used to treat insomnia[a]

Drug	Sleep latency	Sleep continuity[b]	Stage 3/4 NREM sleep amount,%	REM sleep	Other
Trazodone	→	↔ to ↑	↑	↔ amount,% (↓ to ↑ in individual studies)	
Doxepin	→	↑	↔	↓ amount, % of REM; ↑ phasic eye movements (REM density)	*Doxepin, amitriptyline, trimipramine:* ↓ sleep apnea (minor effect); ↔ or ↑ periodic limb movements; ↑restless legs symptoms; may induce eye movements during NREM sleep
Amitriptyline	→	↑	↔	↓ amount, % of REM; ↑ phasic eye movements (REM density)	
Trimipramine	→	↑	↔	↔ amount, %	
Mirtazapine	→	↑	↔	↔	
Melatonin	→	↔ to ↑	↔	↔	
Diphenhydramine	→	↔ to ↑	↔ to ↑	→	
Valerian	→	↔ to ↑	↔ to ↑	↔ to ↑	Inconsistent effects on sleep continuity, Stage 3/4 across studies

Table 2–6. Summary of nonbenzodiazepine drugs used to treat insomnia[a] (*continued*)

Drug	Sleep latency	Sleep continuity[b]	Stage 3/4 NREM sleep amount, %	REM sleep	Other
Gabapentin	↔	↔ to ↑	↑	↔	Reduced periodic limb movements
Tiagabine	↔	↑	↑	↔	Results based on single study
Olanzapine	↔ to ↓	↑	↑	↔ to ↓	Reports of increased periodic limb movements, sleep-eating

Note. REM=rapid eye movement; NREM=non-REM.

[a]Reported effects are based on preponderance of evidence from published studies (see text for details). Many effects are inconsistent between individual studies. ↑ indicates increase from pretreatment baseline; ↓ indicates decrease from pretreatment baseline; ↔ indicates no change from pretreatment baseline.

[b]Sleep continuity refers to the proportion of sleep relative to wakefulness after sleep onset, as reflected by measures such as sleep efficiency. Other indicators of sleep continuity, such as wakefulness after sleep onset or number of awakenings, would have opposite signs. Thus, "↑" indicates improvement in overall sleep continuity.

Sedating tertiary TCAs have polysomnographic effects including reduced sleep latency, reduced wakefulness during sleep, and improved sleep efficiency (Feuillade et al. 1992; Roth et al. 1982; Shipley et al. 1985). Doxepin and amitriptyline also decrease REM sleep amount and increase eye movement activity during REM sleep (Roth et al. 1982; Shipley et al. 1985). Trimipramine, on the other hand, has very few effects on REM sleep. Sedating TCAs have little effect on Stage 3/4 sleep, although some reports show a small increase.

Small studies examining the effects of TCAs in primary insomnia have shown positive effects on both subjective measures and polysomnographic measures such as sleep deficiency (Hajak et al. 2001; Hohagen et al. 1994b).

Mirtazapine

Mirtazapine is a strong serotonin $5-HT_2$ receptor antagonist, with strong antihistamine and α_1-antagonist properties as well. It also antagonizes α_2 noradrenergic receptors (Flores and Schatzberg 2004). Mirtazapine is rapidly absorbed but has a half-life of approximately 20–40 hours (Flores and Schatzberg 2004). Few data are available regarding its effects on sleep. In one study of healthy adults, mirtazapine decreased sleep latency, awakening, and light NREM sleep, and it increased Stage 3/4 sleep (Ruigt et al. 1990). A small study of depressed patients showed similar effects but no change in REM or Stage 3/4 sleep (Winokur et al. 2000). Curiously, mirtazapine has stronger sedative effects at lower doses than at higher doses—presumably because higher doses are associated with more noradrenergic effect.

Antihistamines

Antihistamines are reversible antagonists of CNS histamine H_1 receptors. Histamine, localized in the tuberomammillary nuclei, promotes wakefulness. Sedating antihistamines penetrate the blood-brain barrier readily, whereas nonsedating antihistamines do not. In addition, sedating antihistamines have anticholinergic and serotonergic effects. Diphenhydramine is well absorbed and has a half-life of approximately 4–8 hours. Despite the widespread use of antihistamines, their effects on sleep are not well documented. Clinical trials using doses of 12.5–50 mg have shown subjective improvements in sleep latency, nocturnal awakenings, sleep duration, and sleep quality (Kudo and Kurihara 1990; Meuleman et al. 1987; Rickels et al. 1983). Polysomnographic studies have focused on daytime sedation rather than nighttime sleep effects. In this context, antihistamines produce more rapid sleep onset than placebo, although tolerance to these effects is often seen within a few days (Richardson et al. 2002). Significant side effects of antihistamines include impaired psychomotor performance, cognitive impairment, decreased appetite, and constipation. In older adults, the anticholinergic effects of these medications can be associated with urinary retention.

Melatonin

Melatonin is a hormone normally produced by the pineal gland and secreted exclusively at night. Melatonin production is suppressed by bright light and regulated by the circadian timing system. The most likely effect of melatonin on sleep-wake regulation is its interaction with specific receptors in the suprachiasmatic nucleus of the hypothalamus, the site of the circadian pacemaker. Exogenous melatonin is rapidly absorbed, with peak levels occurring in 20–30 minutes and a very short elimination half-life of 40–60 minutes (DeMuro et al. 2000). Sustained-release preparations can extend the duration of melatonin's effects to several hours.

Melatonin may affect sleep as both a chronobiotic and a hypnotic. As a chronobiotic, melatonin in appropriately timed administration can shift circadian rhythms to an earlier or later phase in a manner that is exactly opposite to that of bright light (see Chapter 7, "Circadian Rhythm Sleep Disorders"). As a hypnotic, melatonin has inconsistent effects. Studies of subjective effects in healthy young adults given melatonin during the daytime, when activity of the suprachiasmatic nucleus is greatest, support its hypnotic efficacy (Cajochen et al. 2003). When given at night, melatonin can decrease subjective sleep latency, although other effects are less consistent. The efficacy of melatonin demonstrated by polysomnographic measures is less well documented.

Some studies have shown increased sleep efficiency, but there is no clear indication of an effect on sleep duration (Olde Rikkert and Rigaud 2001; Sack et al. 1997). Melatonin is generally well tolerated, sedation being its only substantial side effect.

Valerian

Valerian preparations are derived from roots of the plant genus *Valeriana*. The exact amount of various constituents in commercially available preparations is not well described. Likewise, the exact mechanism of valerian preparations is unknown. Some reports suggest GABA-like activity, as indicated by its sedative, anxiolytic, myorelaxant, and possible anticonvulsant effects. Some components of valerian extracts may inhibit GABA metabolism, and interactions with serotonin and adenosine receptors have also been discussed (Houghton 1999; Krystal and Ressler 2001). The pharmacokinetic properties of valerian are not well described because of its multiple constituents.

Sleep studies of valerian show subjective sedative effects, as well as decreased sleep latency and improved sleep quality. Polysomnographic studies have shown a reasonably consistent improvement in sleep latency, but other potential effects, including improved sleep efficiency, increased Stage 3/4 sleep, and reduced Stage 1 sleep, are inconsistent (Balderer and Borbély 1985; Donath et al. 2000). Side effects associated with valerian preparations are typically mild, including sedation, headache, and weakness.

Gabapentin

Gabapentin was initially developed and marketed as an anticonvulsant drug, although it is widely used for treatment of conditions such as chronic pain and insomnia. Its exact mechanism of action is not well understood, although it may promote formation of GABA in the CNS or antagonize N-methyl-D-aspartate receptors (Rose and Kam 2002; Stahl 2000). More recent evidence indicates that gabapentin and a related drug, pregabalin, are ligands for the $\alpha_2\delta$ subunit of voltage-sensitive calcium channels (VSCC). Binding of $\alpha_2\delta$ ligands to activated VSCC reduces calcium influx and reduces neurotransmitter release (Stahl 2004).

Gabapentin has relatively low bioavailability and an elimination half-life of 5–9 hours. Although gabapentin is subjectively sedating, few studies have been conducted on its effects on sleep PSG. A study of epilepsy patients showed decreased awakenings and Stage 1 sleep, as well as increased REM sleep and slow-wave sleep (Foldvary-Schaefer et al. 2002). A study in restless legs syndrome showed similar findings, with increased sleep continuity and increased Stage 3/4 sleep (Garcia-Borreguero et al. 2002). No studies have formally evaluated gabapentin in insomnia.

Tiagabine

Tiagabine is an anticonvulsant drug with a well-defined mechanism of action. It inhibits the GABA transporter GAT-1, reducing GABA reuptake into presynaptic neurons. Tiagabine is rapidly absorbed and metabolized by the cytochrome P450 enzyme CYP3A4, with a half-life of approximately 8 hours. Efficacy studies have not been conducted in insomnia patients. One study in healthy adults demonstrated increased slow-wave sleep and improved sleep efficiency (Mathias et al. 2001). Tiagabine has been associated with new-onset seizures in a small number of patients. The exact frequency of this adverse effect is not known, but it can occur at low doses in patients with no seizure history.

Antipsychotics

Sedating antipsychotics have been used increasingly in the treatment of insomnia, particularly among patients with bipolar and psychotic disorders. The two most commonly used drugs are olanzapine and quetiapine. These drugs have a variety of receptor effects, including antagonist effects at 5-HT$_2$ receptors, dopamine antagonism, and antihistamine effects. Olanzapine is slowly absorbed and has a half-life of 20–54 hours. Quetiapine has a more rapid onset of action, with a peak concentration in 1.5 hours and a half-life of only 6 hours (Baldessarini and Tarazi 2001; Stahl 2000).

A limited number of polysomnographic studies suggest the hypnotic efficacy of olanzapine, which decreases wakefulness, Stage 1 sleep, and REM sleep but increases Stage 3/4 NREM sleep and subjective sleep quality (Lindberg et al. 2002; Sharpley et al. 2000). No published studies are yet available regarding quetiapine as a hypnotic. Consideration should be given to the potentially serious neurological side effects of these medications, as well as their potential effects of weight gain and impaired glucose metabolism.

Clinical Practice Points

Despite the wide array of agents used for the treatment of insomnia, there are no published guidelines regarding the selection of specific drugs, the optimal duration of treatment, the choice of drugs for specific types of insomnia, or strategies to use in cases of partial or complete nonresponsiveness. In most cases of primary insomnia, *a short-acting benzodiazepine receptor agonist is the drug of first choice.* Specific patients may require a benzodiazepine receptor agonist with a longer or shorter duration of action, depending on their pattern of symptoms, sensitivity to medication, and rate of metabolism. For older adults with primary insomnia, smaller doses should be used initially. In cases of partial or no response, substitution or addition of a drug from a different class, usually a sedating antidepressant, is a reasonable choice. Third-line agents would include tiagabine and gabapentin. For patients with concurrent mood or anxiety disorders, BzRA or sedating antidepressants are again appropriate, but only when a primary therapy for the underlying condition, such as psychotherapy or a selective serotonin reuptake inhibitor, is also being used. For patients with known substance use disorders and significant respiratory disease, non-BzRA such as sedating antidepressants should be considered as first-line agents.

In the absence of specific guidelines regarding duration of use, initial treatment should be aimed at *short-term use* of 2–4 weeks. Gradual taper and discontinuation should then be attempted, by decreasing both the dose per administration and the number of doses per week. If longer-term treatment is needed, intermittent use may be preferred to avoid potential tolerance and adverse effects. In some chronic insomnia patients, long-term use of BzRA or other hypnotic drugs is appropriate. Regular monitoring to establish continued efficacy and tolerability of side effects is essential.

Behavioral treatments should be considered and utilized whenever possible, even in patients receiving pharmacotherapy. Long-term efficacy is better established for behavioral treatments than for pharmacologic treatments, and it seems prudent to avoid medications and their potential side effects when such efficacious other treatments are available.

Summary

Insomnia is a prevalent health complaint that is strongly associated with psychiatric and medical disorders. Recent studies have suggested that increased CNS arousal may be a common final pathway for different subtypes of insomnia. In addition, cognitive and behavioral factors often play an important role. The assessment of insomnia rests on a detailed and accurate clinical history, supplemented by sleep diaries and other tools. Efficacious treatments for insomnia include behavioral and cognitive-behavioral therapy and pharmacotherapy with benzodiazepine receptor agonists and, potentially, antidepressant medications. Although a wide number of other medications have been used to treat insomnia, their efficacy remains to be demonstrated. Insomnia has a significant effect on quality of life and daytime function, and treatment can result in improved functioning.

References

Agargun MY, Kara H, Solmaz M: Subjective sleep quality and suicidality in patients with major depression. J Psychiatr Res 31:377–381, 1997

Allard J, Artero S, Ritchie K: Consumption of psychotropic medication in the elderly: a re-evaluation of its effect on cognitive performance. Int J Geriatr Psychiatry 18:874–878, 2003

American Academy of Sleep Medicine: International Classification of Sleep Disorders, 2nd Edition. Westchester, IL, American Academy of Sleep Medicine (in press)

American Psychiatric Association: Diagnostic and Statistical Manual of Mental Disorders, 4th Edition, Text Revision. Washington, DC, American Psychiatric Association, 2000

American Sleep Disorders Association: International Classification of Sleep Disorders, Revised: Diagnostic and Coding Manual. Rochester, MN, American Sleep Disorders Association, 1997

Asnis GM, Chakraburtty A, DuBoff EA, et al: Zolpidem for persistent insomnia in SSRI-treated depressed patients. J Clin Psychiatry 60:668–676, 1999

Attenburrow ME, Dowling BA, Sharpley AL, et al: Case-control study of evening melatonin concentration in primary insomnia. BMJ 312:1263–1264, 1996

Balderer G, Borbély AA: Effect of valerian on human sleep. Psychopharmacology (Berl) 87:406–409, 1985

Baldessarini RJ, Tarazi FI: Drugs and the treatment of anxiety disorders: psychosis and mania, in Goodman and Gilman's The Pharmacological Basis of Therapeutics. Edited by Hardman JG, Limbird LE. New York, McGraw-Hill, 2001, pp 485–520

Bateson AN: The benzodiazepine site of the $GABA_A$ receptor: an old target with new potential? Sleep Med 1 (5 suppl):S9–S15, 2004

Bonnet MH, Arand DL: 24-Hour metabolic rate in insomniacs and matched normal sleepers. Sleep 18:581–588, 1995

Bonnet MH, Arand DL: Hyperarousal and insomnia. Sleep Med Rev 1:97–108, 1997a

Bonnet MH, Arand DL: Physiological activation in patients with sleep state misperception. Psychosom Med 59:533–540, 1997b

Bootzin RR, Nicassio PM: Behavioral treatments of insomnia, in Progress in Behavior Modification, Vol 6. Edited by Hersen M, Eisler RE, Miller PM. New York, Academic Press, 1978, pp 1–45

Brassington GS, King AC, Bliwise DL: Sleep problems as a risk factor for falls in a sample of community-dwelling adults aged 64–99 years. J Am Geriatr Soc 48:1234–1240, 2000

Breslau N, Roth T, Rosenthal L, et al: Sleep disturbance and psychiatric disorders: a longitudinal epidemiological study of young adults. Biol Psychiatry 39:411–418, 1996

Brower KJ, Aldrich MS, Robinson EA, et al: Insomnia, self-medication, and relapse to alcoholism. Am J Psychiatry 158:399–404, 2001

Buysse DJ, Reynolds CF 3rd, Hauri PJ, et al: Diagnostic concordance for DSM-IV sleep disorders: a report from the APA/NIMH DSM-IV field trial. Am J Psychiatry 151:1351–1360, 1994

Buysse DJ, Tu XM, Cherry CR, et al: Pretreatment REM sleep and subjective sleep quality distinguish depressed psychotherapy remitters and nonremitters. Biol Psychiatry 45:205–213, 1999

Cajochen C, Kräuchi K, Wirz-Justice A: Role of melatonin in the regulation of human circadian rhythms and sleep. J Neuroendocrinol 15:432–437, 2003

Camacho ME, Morin CM: The effect of temazepam on respiration in elderly insomniacs with mild sleep apnea. Sleep 18:644–645, 1995

Chang PP, Ford DE, Mead LA, et al: Insomnia in young men and subsequent depression: the Johns Hopkins Precursors Study. Am J Epidemiol 146:105–114, 1997

Coull JT: Neural correlates of attention and arousal: insights from electrophysiology, functional neuroimaging and psychopharmacology. Prog Neurobiol 55:343–361, 1998

Cumming RG, Le Couteur DG: Benzodiazepines and risk of hip fractures in older people: a review of the evidence. CNS Drugs 17:825–837, 2003

Curran HV, Collins R, Fletcher S, et al: Older adults and withdrawal from benzodiazepine hypnotics in general practice: effects on cognitive function, sleep, mood and quality of life. Psychol Med 33:1223–1237, 2003

Currie SR, Wilson KG, Pontefract AJ, et al: Cognitive-behavioral treatment of insomnia secondary to chronic pain. J Consult Clin Psychol 68:407–416, 2000

D'Ambrosio C, Bowman T, Mohsenin V: Quality of life in patients with obstructive sleep apnea: effect of nasal continuous positive airway pressure—a prospective study. Chest 115:123–129, 1999

DeMuro RL, Nafziger AN, Blask DE, et al: The absolute bioavailability of oral melatonin. J Clin Pharmacol 40:781–784, 2000

Donath F, Quispe S, Diefenbach K, et al: Critical evaluation of the effect of valerian extract on sleep structure and sleep quality. Pharmacopsychiatry 33:47–53, 2000

Edinger JD, Sampson WS: A primary care "friendly" cognitive behavior insomnia therapy. Sleep 26:177–182, 2003

Espie CA, Inglis SJ, Harvey L: Predicting clinically significant response to cognitive behavior therapy for chronic insomnia in general medical practice: analyses of outcome data at 12 months posttreatment. J Consult Clin Psychol 69:58–66, 2001

Feuillade P, Pringuey D, Belugou JL: Trimipramine: acute and lasting effects on sleep in healthy and major depressive subjects. J Affect Disord 24:135–145, 1992

Flores BH, Schatzberg AF: Mirtazapine, in The American Psychiatric Publishing Textbook of Psychopharmacology, 3rd Edition. Edited by Schatzberg AF, Nemeroff CB. Washington, DC, American Psychiatric Publishing, 2004, pp 341–347

Foldvary-Schaefer N, De Leon Sanchez I, Karafa M, et al: Gabapentin increases slow-wave sleep in normal adults. Epilepsia 43:1493–1497, 2002

Foley DJ, Monjan A, Simonsick EM, et al: Incidence and remission of insomnia among elderly adults: an epidemiologic study of 6,800 persons over three years. Sleep 22:S366–S372, 1999

Garcia-Borreguero D, Larrosa O, de la Llave Y, et al: Treatment of restless legs syndrome with gabapentin: a double-blind, cross-over study. Neurology 59:1573–1579, 2002

Golden RN, Dawkins K, Nicholas L: Trazodone and nefazodone, in The American Psychiatric Textbook of Psychopharmacology, 3rd Edition. Edited by Schatzberg AF, Nemeroff CB. Washington, DC, American Psychiatric Publishing, 2004, pp 315–325

Griffiths RR, Weerts EM: Benzodiazepine self-administration in humans and laboratory animals: implications for problems of long-term use and abuse. Psychopharmacology (Berl) 134:1–37, 1997

Gross RT, Borkovec TD: Effects of a cognitive intrusion manipulation on the sleep-onset latency of good sleepers. Behav Ther 13:112–116, 1982

Hajak G, Rodenbeck A, Staedt J, et al: Nocturnal plasma melatonin levels in patients suffering from chronic primary insomnia. J Pineal Res 19:116–122, 1995

Hajak G, Rodenbeck A, Voderholzer U, et al: Doxepin in the treatment of primary insomnia: a placebo-controlled, double-blind, polysomnographic study. J Clin Psychiatry 62:453–463, 2001

Harvey AG: A cognitive model of insomnia. Behav Res Ther 40:869–893, 2002

Hatoum HT, Kong SX, Kania CM, et al: Insomnia, health-related quality of life and healthcare resource consumption: a study of managed-care organisation enrollees. Pharmacoeconomics 14:629–637, 1998

Hauri PJ: Case Studies in Insomnia. New York, Kluwer Academic, 1991

Hohagen F, Kappler C, Schramm E, et al: Sleep onset insomnia, sleep maintaining insomnia and insomnia with early morning awakening: temporal stability of subtypes in a longitudinal study on general practice attenders. Sleep 17:551–554, 1994a

Hohagen F, Montero RF, Weiss E, et al: Treatment of primary insomnia with trimipramine: an alternative to benzodiazepine hypnotics? Eur Arch Psychiatry Clin Neurosci 244:65–72, 1994b

Holbrook AM, Crowther R, Lotter A, et al: Meta-analysis of benzodiazepine use in the treatment of insomnia. CMAJ 162:225–233, 2000

Houghton PJ: The scientific basis for the reputed activity of valerian. J Pharm Pharmacol 51:505–512, 1999

Jacobson E: Progressive Relaxation: A Physiological and Clinical Investigation of Muscular States and Their Significance in Psychology and Medical Practice, 3rd Revised Edition. Chicago, IL, University of Chicago Press, 1974

James SP, Mendelson WB: The use of trazodone as a hypnotic: a critical review. J Clin Psychiatry 65:752–755, 2004

Kappler C, Hohagen F: Psychosocial aspects of insomnia: results of a study in general practice. Eur Arch Psychiatry Clin Neurosci 253:49–52, 2003

Karlsen KH, Larsen JP, Tandberg E, et al: Influence of clinical and demographic variables on quality of life in patients with Parkinson's disease. J Neurol Neurosurg Psychiatry 66:431–435, 1999

Katz DA, McHorney CA: Clinical correlates of insomnia in patients with chronic illness. Arch Intern Med 158:1099–1107, 1998

Katz DA, McHorney CA: The relationship between insomnia and health-related quality of life in patients with chronic illness. J Fam Pract 51:229–235, 2002

Koski K, Luukinen H, Laippala P, et al: Risk factors for major injurious falls among the home-dwelling elderly by functional abilities: a prospective population-based study. Gerontology 44:232–238, 1998

Krystal AD, Ressler I: The use of valerian in neuropsychiatry. CNS Spectr 6:841–847, 2001

Krystal AD, Edinger JD, Wohlgemuth WK, et al: NREM sleep EEG frequency spectral correlates of sleep complaints in primary insomnia subtypes. Sleep 25:630–640, 2002

Krystal AD, Walsh JK, Laska E, et al: Sustained efficacy of eszopiclone over 6 months of nightly treatment: results of a randomized, double-blind, placebo-controlled study in adults with chronic insomnia. Sleep 26:793–799, 2003

Kudo Y, Kurihara M: Clinical evaluation of diphenhydramine hydrochloride for the treatment of insomnia in psychiatric patients: a double-blind study. J Clin Pharmacol 30:1041–1048, 1990

Lacks P, Morin CM: Recent advances in the assessment and treatment of insomnia. J Consult Clin Psychol 60:586–594, 1992

Léger D, Scheuermaier K, Philip P, et al: SF-36: evaluation of quality of life in severe and mild insomniacs compared with good sleepers. Psychosom Med 63:49–55, 2001

Léger D, Guilleminault C, Bader G, et al: Medical and socio-professional impact of insomnia. Sleep 25:625–629, 2002

Lichstein KL, Wilson NM, Johnson CT: Psychological treatment of secondary insomnia. Psychol Aging 15:232–240, 2000

Lindberg N, Virkkunen M, Tani P, et al: Effect of a single-dose of olanzapine on sleep in healthy females and males. Int Clin Psychopharmacol 17:177–184, 2002

Lofaso F, Goldenberg F, Thebault C, et al: Effect of zopiclone on sleep, night-time ventilation, and daytime vigilance in upper airway resistance syndrome. Eur Respir J 10:2573–2577, 1997

Mathias S, Wetter TC, Steiger A, et al: The GABA uptake inhibitor tiagabine promotes slow-wave sleep in normal elderly subjects. Neurobiol Aging 22:247–253, 2001

McCall WV, Reboussin BA, Cohen W: Subjective measurement of insomnia and quality of life in depressed inpatients. J Sleep Res 9:43–48, 2000

McCurry SM, Ancoli-Israel S: Sleep dysfunction in Alzheimer's disease and other dementias. Curr Treat Options Neurol 5:261–272, 2003

Mendelson WB: Long-term follow-up of chronic insomnia. Sleep 18:698–701, 1995

Merica H, Gaillard JM: The EEG of the sleep onset period in insomnia: a discriminant analysis. Physiol Behav 52:199–204, 1992

Merica H, Blois R, Gaillard JM: Spectral characteristics of sleep EEG in chronic insomnia. Eur J Neurosci 10:1826–1834, 1998

Meuleman JR, Nelson RC, Clark RL: Evaluation of temazepam and diphenhydramine as hypnotics in a nursing-home population. Drug Intell Clin Pharm 21:716–720, 1987

Mimeault V, Morin CM: Self-help treatment for insomnia: bibliotherapy with and without professional guidance. J Consult Clin Psychol 67:511–519, 1999

Mohler H, Fritschy J, Rudolph U: A new benzodiazepine pharmacology. J Pharmacol Exp Ther 300:2–8, 2002

Montgomery P, Dennis J: Cognitive behavioural interventions for sleep problems in adults aged 60+. Cochrane Database Syst Rev (1): CD003161, 2003

Moos RH, Cronkite RC: Symptom-based predictors of a 10-year chronic course of treated depression. J Nerv Ment Dis 187:360–368, 1999

Morin CM: Insomnia: Psychological Assessment and Management. New York, Guilford, 1993

Morin CM, Kowatch RA, Wade JB: Behavioral management of sleep disturbances secondary to chronic pain. J Behav Ther Exp Psychiatry 20:295–302, 1989

Morin CM, Culbert JP, Schwartz SM: Nonpharmacological interventions for insomnia: a meta-analysis of treatment efficacy. Am J Psychiatry 151:1172–1180, 1994

Morin CM, Hauri PJ, Espie CA, et al: Nonpharmacologic treatment of chronic insomnia. Sleep 22:1135–1156, 1999

Moul DE, Nofzinger EA, Pilkonis PA, et al: Symptom reports in severe chronic insomnia. Sleep 25:553–563, 2002

Moul DE, Hall M, Pilkonis PA, et al: Self-report measures of insomnia adults: rationales, choices, and needs. Sleep Med Rev 8:177–198, 2004

Murtagh DR, Greenwood KM: Identifying effective psychological treatments for insomnia: a meta-analysis. J Consult Clin Psychol 63:79–89, 1995

Nelson JC: Tricyclic and tetracyclic drugs, in The American Psychiatric Publishing Textbook of Psychopharmacology, 3rd Edition. Edited by Schatzberg AF, Nemeroff CB. Washington, DC, American Psychiatric Publishing, 2004, pp 207–230

Nofzinger EA, Price JC, Meltzer CC, et al: Towards a neurobiology of dysfunctional arousal in depression: the relationship between beta EEG power and regional cerebral glucose metabolism during NREM sleep. Psychiatry Res 98:71–91, 2000

Nofzinger EA, Buysse DJ, Germain A, et al: Functional neuroimaging evidence for hyperarousal in insomnia. Am J Psychiatry 161:2126–2128, 2004

Nowell PD, Mazumdar S, Buysse DJ, et al: Benzodiazepines and zolpidem for chronic insomnia: a meta-analysis of treatment efficacy. JAMA 278:2170–2177, 1997

Ohayon MM: Prevalence of DSM-IV diagnostic criteria of insomnia: distinguishing insomnia related to mental disorders from sleep disorders. J Psychiatr Res 31:333–346, 1997

Ohayon MM: Epidemiology of insomnia: what we know and what we still need to learn. Sleep Med Rev 6:97–111, 2002

Ohayon MM, Guilleminault C: Epidemiology of sleep disorders, in Sleep Disorders Medicine: Basic Science, Technical Considerations, and Clinical Aspects, 2nd Edition. Edited by Chokroverty S. Boston, MA, Butterworth-Heinemann, 1999, pp 301–316

Olde Rikkert MG, Rigaud AS: Melatonin in elderly patients with insomnia: a systematic review. Z Gerontol Geriatr 34:491–497, 2001

Oswald I, French C, Adam K, et al: Benzodiazepine hypnotics remain effective for 24 weeks. Br Med J (Clin Res Ed) 284:860–863, 1982

Parrino L, Terzano MG: Polysomnographic effects of hypnotic drugs: a review. Psychopharmacology (Berl) 126:1–16, 1996

Parrino L, Spaggiari MC, Boselli M, et al: Clinical and polysomnographic effects of trazodone CR in chronic insomnia associated with dysthymia. Psychopharmacology (Berl) 116:389–395, 1994

Perlis ML, Giles DE, Buysse DJ, et al: Self-reported sleep disturbance as a prodromal symptom in recurrent depression. J Affect Disord 42:209–212, 1997a

Perlis ML, Giles DE, Mendelson WB, et al: Psychophysiological insomnia: the behavioural model and a neurocognitive perspective. J Sleep Res 6:179–188, 1997b

Perlis ML, Smith MT, Andrews PJ, et al: Beta/gamma EEG activity in patients with primary and secondary insomnia and good sleeper controls. Sleep 24:110–117, 2001

Perlis ML, McCall WV, Krystal AD, et al: Long-term, non-nightly administration of zolpidem in the treatment of patients with primary insomnia. J Clin Psychiatry 65:1128–1137, 2004

Powell NB, Schechtman KB, Riley RW, et al: Sleepy driving: accidents and injury. Otolaryngol Head Neck Surg 126:217–227, 2002

Reynolds CF 3rd, Frank E, Houck PR, et al: Which elderly patients with remitted depression remain well with continued interpersonal psychotherapy after discontinuation of antidepressant medication? Am J Psychiatry 154:958–962, 1997

Richardson GS, Roehrs TA, Rosenthal L, et al: Tolerance to daytime sedative effects of H_1 antihistamines. J Clin Psychopharmacol 22:511–515, 2002

Rickels K, Morris RJ, Newman H, et al: Diphenhydramine in insomniac family practice patients: a double-blind study. J Clin Pharmacol 23:234–242, 1983

Riemann D, Voderholzer U: Primary insomnia: a risk factor to develop depression? J Affect Disord 76:255–259, 2003

Rodenbeck A, Huether G, Ruther E, et al: Interactions between evening and nocturnal cortisol secretion and sleep parameters in patients with severe chronic primary insomnia. Neurosci Lett 324:159–163, 2002

Roehrs T, Merlotti L, Zorick F, et al: Sedative, memory, and performance effects of hypnotics. Psychopharmacology (Berl) 116:130–134, 1994

Rose MA, Kam PC: Gabapentin: pharmacology and its use in pain management. Anaesthesia 57:451–462, 2002

Roth T, Zorick F, Wittig R, et al: The effects of doxepin HCl on sleep and depression. J Clin Psychiatry 43:366–368, 1982

Ruigt GS, Kemp B, Groenhout CM, et al: Effect of the antidepressant Org 3770 on human sleep. Eur J Clin Pharmacol 38:551–554, 1990

Rybarczyk B, Lopez M, Benson R, et al: Efficacy of two behavioral treatment programs for comorbid geriatric insomnia. Psychol Aging 17:288–298, 2002

Sack RL, Hughes RJ, Edgar DM, et al: Sleep-promoting effects of melatonin: at what dose, in whom, under what conditions, and by what mechanisms? Sleep 20:908–915, 1997

Sadeh A, Acebo C: The role of actigraphy in sleep medicine. Sleep Med Rev 6:113–124, 2002

Saletu M, Anderer P, Saletu-Zyhlarz G, et al: Restless legs syndrome (RLS) and periodic limb movement disorder (PLMD): acute placebo-controlled sleep laboratory studies with clonazepam. Eur Neuropsychopharmacol 11:153–161, 2001

Saletu-Zyhlarz G, Abu-Bakr M, Anderer P, et al: Insomnia in depression: differences in objective and subjective sleep awakening quality to normal controls and acute effects of trazodone. Prog Neuropsychopharmacol Biol Psychiatry 26:249–260, 2002

Sateia MJ, Doghramji K, Hauri PJ, et al: Evaluation of chronic insomnia: an American Academy of Sleep Medicine review. Sleep 23:243–308, 2000

Scharf MB, Roth T, Vogel GW, et al: A multicenter, placebo-controlled study evaluating zolpidem in the treatment of chronic insomnia. J Clin Psychiatry 55:192–199, 1994

Sharpley AL, Vassallo CM, Cowen PJ: Olanzapine increases slow-wave sleep: evidence for blockade of central 5-HT(2C) receptors in vivo. Biol Psychiatry 47:468–470, 2000

Shipley JE, Kupfer DJ, Griffin SJ, et al: Comparison of effects of desipramine and amitriptyline on EEG sleep of depressed patients. Psychopharmacology (Berl) 85:14–22, 1985

Simeit R, Deck R, Conta-Marx B: Sleep management training for cancer patients with insomnia. Support Care Cancer 12:176–183, 2004

Simon GE, Von Korff M: Prevalence, burden, and treatment of insomnia in primary care. Am J Psychiatry 154:1417–1423, 1997

Smith MT, Perlis ML, Chengazi VU, et al: Neuroimaging of NREM sleep in primary insomnia: a Tc-99-HMPAO single photon emission computed tomography study. Sleep 25:325–335, 2002a

Smith MT, Perlis ML, Park A, et al: Comparative meta-analysis of pharmacotherapy and behavior therapy for persistent insomnia. Am J Psychiatry 159:5–11, 2002b

Smith WT, Londborg PD, Glaudin V, et al: Is extended clonazepam cotherapy of fluoxetine effective for outpatients with major depression? J Affect Disord 70:251–259, 2002

Sok SR, Erlen JA, Kim KB: Effects of acupuncture therapy on insomnia. J Adv Nurs 44:375–384, 2003

Soldatos CR, Dikeos DG, Whitehead A: Tolerance and rebound insomnia with rapidly eliminated hypnotics: a meta-analysis of sleep laboratory studies. Int Clin Psychopharmacol 14:287–303, 1999

Spielman AJ, Caruso LS, Glovinsky PB: A behavioral perspective on insomnia treatment. Psychiatr Clin North Am 10:541–553, 1987

Stahl SM: Essential Pharmacology: Neuroscientific Basis and Practical Applications, 2nd Edition. New York, Cambridge University Press, 2000

Stahl SM: Mechanism of action of alpha2delta ligands: voltage sensitive calcium channel (VSCC) modulators. J Clin Psychiatry 65:1033–1034, 2004

Strom L, Pettersson R, Andersson G: Internet-based treatment for insomnia: a controlled evaluation. J Consult Clin Psychol 72:113–120, 2004

Thomas RE: Benzodiazepine use and motor vehicle accidents: systematic review of reported association. Can Fam Physician 44:799–808, 1998

van Bemmel AL, Havermans RG, van Diest R: Effects of trazodone on EEG sleep and clinical state in major depression. Psychopharmacology (Berl) 107:569–574, 1992

Vermeeren A: Residual effects of hypnotics: epidemiology and clinical implications. CNS Drugs 18:297–328, 2004

Vgontzas AN, Bixler EO, Lin HM, et al: Chronic insomnia is associated with nyctohemeral activation of the hypothalamic-pituitary-adrenal axis: clinical implications. J Clin Endocrinol Metab 86:3787–3794, 2001

Vollrath M, Wicki W, Angst J: The Zurich study, VIII. Insomnia: association with depression, anxiety, somatic syndromes, and course of insomnia. Eur Arch Psychiatry Neurol Sci 239:113–124, 1989

Walsh JK: Drugs used to treat insomnia in 2002: regulatory-based rather than evidence-based medicine. Sleep 1441–1442, 2004

Walsh JK, Engelhardt CL: The direct economic costs of insomnia in the United States for 1995. Sleep 22:S386–S393, 1999

Walsh JK, Erman M, Erwin CW, et al: Subjective hypnotic efficacy of trazodone and zolpidem in DSM-III-R primary insomnia. Hum Psychopharmacol 13:191–198, 1998

Walsh JK, Schweitzer PK: Ten-year trends in the pharmacological treatment of insomnia. Sleep 22:371–375, 1999

Walsh JK, Roth T, Randazzo A, et al: Eight weeks of non-nightly use of zolpidem for primary insomnia. Sleep 23:1087–1096, 2000a

Walsh JK, Vogel GW, Scharf M, et al: A five week, polysomnographic assessment of zaleplon 10 mg for the treatment of primary insomnia. Sleep Med 1:41–49, 2000b

Winokur A, Sateia MJ, Hayes JB, et al: Acute effects of mirtazapine on sleep continuity and sleep architecture in depressed patients: a pilot study. Biol Psychiatry 48:75–78, 2000

Woods JH, Winger G: Current benzodiazepine issues. Psychopharmacology (Berl) 118:107–115, 1995

Woolfolk RL, McNulty TF: Relaxation treatment for insomnia: a component analysis. J Consult Clin Psychol 51:495–503, 1983

World Health Organization: International Statistical Classification of Diseases and Related Health Problems, 10th Revision. Geneva, World Health Organization, 1992

Chapter 3

Sleep Apnea

Patrick J. Strollo, Jr., M.D.
Nilesh B. Davé, M.D., M.P.H.

The focus of this review will be on the diagnosis and management of obstructive sleep apnea/hypopnea syndrome (OSAH) in adults. OSAH is a common clinical problem that is associated with significant morbidity and mortality. It is relatively easily diagnosed and treated. In this chapter we will discuss the spectrum of obstructive sleep-disordered breathing, with particular attention to how it affects psychiatric practice.

Definitions

The clinical condition of obstructive sleep-disordered breathing includes obstructive apnea (OSA) and obstructive hypopnea. An *obstructive apnea* is defined as a lack of airflow measured at the nose and mouth for 10 seconds or longer during sleep, despite ongoing effort to breathe. This is usually associated with a decrease in the oxyhemoglobin saturation and a change in the electroencephalogram (EEG) indicating arousal from sleep. An *obstructive hypopnea* is defined as a decrease in airflow (generally ≥30%) at the nose and mouth despite ongoing effort to breathe. These events are also associated with a decrease in the oxyhemoglobin saturation and a change in the EEG indicating arousal from sleep (Strollo and Rogers 1996) (Figure 3–1 and Figure 3–2).

Various methods are available to measure airflow cessation (apnea) and limitation (hypopnea) during sleep. In 1999, the American Academy of Sleep Medicine examined the evidence on the measuring of sleep-disordered breathing events and attempted to establish a consensus for the definitions of obstructive sleep apnea and obstructive sleep hypopnea. Apneas in adults are easily identified

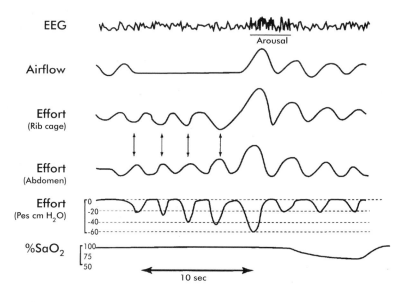

Figure 3–1. Obstructive apnea.

Increasing ventilatory effort is seen in the rib cage, the abdomen, and the level of esophageal pressure (measured with an esophageal balloon), despite lack of oronasal airflow. Arousal on the electroencephalogram (EEG) is associated with increasing ventilatory effort, as indicated by the esophageal pressure. Oxyhemoglobin desaturation follows the termination of apnea. Note that during apnea, the movements of the rib cage and the abdomen (Effort) are in opposite directions (arrows) as a result of attempts to breathe against a closed airway. Once the airway opens in response to arousal, rib cage and abdominal movements become synchronous. Pes=esophageal pressure.
Source. Adapted from Strollo and Rogers 1996.

even with simple monitoring devices such as thermal sensors (thermisters or thermocouples). This is not the case for airflow limitation (hypopnea). The accuracy of measurement of airflow limitation can be substantially influenced by the method of measurement.

On polysomnography (PSG), both apneas and hypopneas are commonly associated with changes on the EEG as a marker of sleep disruption. However, the intrarater and interrater reliability for visual scoring of arousals is variable. Including arousal criteria when scoring hypopneas has not led to an increase in precision (Tsai et al. 1999). This finding has led to a refined operational definition of sleep hypopnea. In current clinical practice, hypopneas

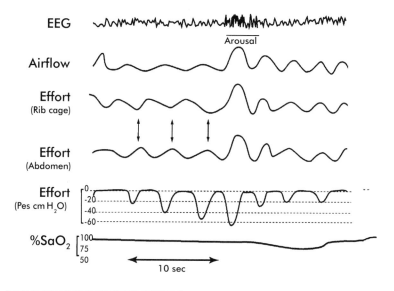

Figure 3–2. Obstructive hypopnea.

Decreased airflow is associated with increasing ventilatory effort (reflected by the esophageal pressure) and subsequent arousal on the electroencephalogram (EEG). Rib cage and abdominal movements are in opposite directions during hypopnea (arrows), reflecting increasingly difficult breathing against a partially closed airway. Rib cage and abdominal movements become synchronous after arousal produces airway opening. Oxyhemoglobin desaturation follows the termination of hypopnea. Pes = esophageal pressure.
Source. Adapted from Strollo and Rogers 1996.

that are associated with ≥4% desaturations, without arousal criteria, are accepted as physiologically significant events. Neurocognitive and cardiovascular outcomes identified primarily in the Sleep Heart Health Study have provided the rationale for combining apneas and hypopneas to produce an apnea-hypopnea index (AHI) to rate syndrome severity (American Academy of Sleep Medicine 1999; Gottlieb et al. 1999; Shahar et al. 2001).

Mild OSA is defined as an AHI of 5–15 events per hour of sleep. Moderate OSA is defined as an AHI of 15–30 events per hour of sleep. Severe OSA is defined as an AHI of greater than 30 events per hour of sleep. For the condition to meet "syndrome" criteria, the clinical complaint of disturbed sleep and/or daytime sleepiness should be present (Table 3–1).

Table 3–1. International Classification of Sleep Disorders diagnostic criteria for obstructive sleep apnea/hypopnea syndrome (580.53–0)

Definition: Obstructive sleep apnea/hypopnea syndrome is characterized by repetitive episodes of upper airway obstruction (apnea or hypopnea) that occur during sleep, usually associated with a reduction in blood oxygenation

Diagnostic criteria
    A. A complaint of excessive sleepiness or insomnia
    B. Frequent episodes of obstructed breathing during sleep
    C. Associated features
        a. Loud snoring
        b. Morning headaches
        c. Dry mouth upon awakening
        d. Chest retraction during sleep (children)
    D. Polysomnographic findings
        a. An apnea-hypopnea index (AHI) of ≥ 5 and one of the following:
            i. Frequent arousals from sleep associated with apneas/hypopneas
            ii. Bradytachycardia
            iii. Oxyhemoglobin desaturation associated with the apneic/hypopneic episodes
            iv. A mean sleep latency of <10 minutes on multiple sleep latency testing
    E. Can be associated with other medical disorders (e.g., tonsillar hypertrophy)
    F. Other sleep disorders can be present (e.g., narcolepsy, periodic limb movements)

Minimum criteria: A plus B plus C

Severity criteria
    Mild: AHI 5–15
    Moderate: AHI 15–30
    Severe: AHI >30

Source. American Academy of Sleep Medicine 1999.

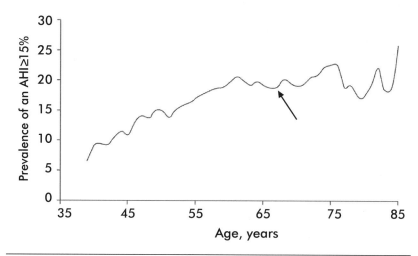

Figure 3–3. Effect of age on prevalence of obstructive sleep apnea/hypopnea.

The smoothed plot (5-year moving average) depicting the prevalence, by age, of an apnea-hypopnea index (AHI) ≥15. The arrow denotes a plateau in the prevalence that occurs at approximately age 65.

Source. From Young T et al: "Predictors of Sleep-Disordered Breathing in Community-Dwelling Adults: The Sleep Heart Health Study." *Archives of Internal Medicine* 162:893–900, 2002. ©2002 American Medical Association. All rights reserved.

Epidemiology

The epidemiology of OSAH has been well described in North America and Europe (Young et al. 2002a). In predominantly Caucasian middle-aged cohorts, the prevalence of OSAH (defined as AHI ≥10 plus symptoms of daytime sleepiness and/or hypertension) is approximately 5%.

Clinical studies indicate an increased risk in men, with a prevalence ratio of 3.3:1 compared with women (Bixler et al. 2001). The prevalence of OSAH in middle-aged individuals has been reported to be 4% for men and 2% for women (Young et al. 1993).

Menopause appears to increase the risk of OSAH, as does obesity. In a central Pennsylvania population, Bixler et al. (2001) reported a prevalence of 2.7% for OSAH in postmenopausal women without hormonal replacement therapy, as opposed to 0.6% in the premenopausal population. Preliminary data suggest that the prevalence of OSAH may be higher in the African American than in the Caucasian population (Ancoli-Israel et al. 1995).

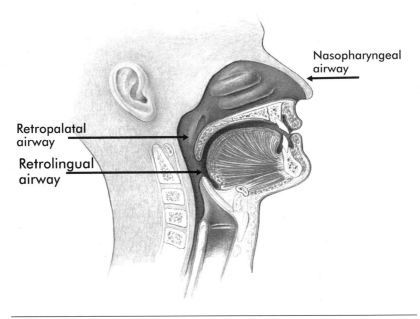

Figure 3–4. Cross-sectional view of the upper airway depicting the potential sites of airway instability (arrows).

In a longitudinal family study, Redline's group reported a 5-year incidence of 7.5% for mild OSAH (AHI $\geq 10 < 15$) and 16% for moderate to severe OSAH (AHI ≥ 15) (Tishler et al. 2003). Advancing age and increasing weight independently increase the risk of OSAH (Young et al. 2002a). The age effect appears to plateau after age 65 (Figure 3–3), implying that there may be an increase in mortality in middle age, or possibly remission of OSAH in the elderly population (Young et al. 2002b).

Pathophysiology

The upper airway in humans is able to perform a variety of complex functions, including breathing, swallowing, and speaking. This is possible in part because of the lack of rigid support from bone or cartilaginous tissue in the retropalatal and retrolingual airway (Figure 3–4). When increased negative intrathoracic pressure results in a suction force applied to a small, compliant upper airway, narrowing (hypopnea) or closure (apnea) may oc-

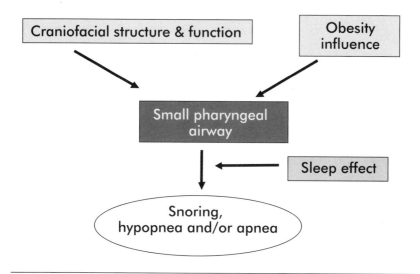

Figure 3–5. Pathogenesis of obstructive sleep apnea/hypopnea. General factors influencing the development of obstructive sleep apnea/hypopnea in patients who are at risk (i.e., small pharyngeal airway).

cur. This is frequently accompanied by vibration of these structures that produces snoring sounds.

The primary cause for airway closure during sleep is a small airway. Craniofacial structure and function, in addition to obesity, are the major determinants of a small airway in adults. Individuals with OSAH are able to maintain airway patency during wakefulness. During the transition from the wake to the sleeping state, muscle tone decreases and snoring, airway narrowing, and/or closure may occur in individuals with a "vulnerable airway" (Figure 3–5).

The uniform stimulus for resumption of normal breathing is a ventilatory-related arousal from sleep (Gleeson et al. 1990). The arousal is usually identifiable on the electroencephalographic channel when sleep and breathing are measured in the laboratory. The ventilatory-related arousal may be precipitated by increased airway resistance (usually associated with snoring), hypopnea, or apnea.

Other important physiological perturbations occur in conjunction with the sleep-disordered breathing events. Struggling against a partially or completely closed airway is associated with increased intrathoracic pressure, hypoventilation, and increased vagal tone. The ensuing arousal is accompanied by augmentation of sympathetic tone. These phenomena have acute and chronic effects on cardiovascular function. Acute changes are manifested as bradycardia followed by tachycardia (i.e., heart rate variability). Over time, sympathetic tone is upregulated not only nocturnally but also diurnally (Somers et al. 1995).

Intermittent hypoxemia is a hallmark of OSAH. Recent data suggest that the ischemia-reperfusion associated with intermittent hypoxemia results in transcription and translation of biomarkers of oxidative stress and subsequent endothelial dysfunction (Lavie 2003). A number of these biomarkers, such as C-reactive protein and interleukin-6, have been linked to risk and progression of cardiovascular disease in addition to altered metabolic function (see next section).

Consequences

OSAH is associated with significant comorbidities that result from the altered nocturnal physiology. These comorbidities can be broadly grouped into three categories: cardiovascular, metabolic, and neurocognitive complications (Table 3–2). Observational studies have established a relationship between apnea-hypopnea severity and these conditions. Data now exist that demonstrate that adequate treatment of OSAH, primarily with positive pressure, favorably affects these comorbidities (see "Therapy" section below). Although one or all of the comorbidities may affect an individual patient, each category will be discussed separately for clarity.

Cardiovascular Complications

The normal cardiovascular response to sleep, including a decrease in blood pressure and heart rate, is negatively affected in OSAH. Acute and chronic physiological effects related to sleep-disordered breathing occur.

The repetitive bursts of sympathetic activity triggered by sleep-disordered breathing events adversely affect nocturnal blood pressure and heart rate. Over time, a profound toll is taken on the cardiovascular system. Risk is increased for diurnal sys-

Table 3–2. Comorbidities associated with obstructive sleep apnea/hypopnea syndrome

Cardiovascular complications
    Nocturnal dysrhythmias
        Bradydysrhythmias
        Atrial fibrillation
    Nocturnal hypertension
    Diurnal hypertension
    Pulmonary hypertension
    Congestive heart failure
    Myocardial infarction
    Stroke

Metabolic complications
    Leptin resistance
    Insulin resistance

Neurocognitive complications
    Daytime sleepiness
    Motor vehicle accidents
    Work-related accidents
    Impaired neuropsychological function
    Impaired quality of life

temic hypertension, diurnal pulmonary hypertension, atrial dysrhythmias, heart failure (systolic and diastolic), myocardial infarction, and stroke.

Cross-sectional observational studies suggest a relationship between apnea-hypopnea severity and cardiovascular complications (Peppard et al. 2000b; Shahar et al. 2001). The best evidence linking OSAH to cardiovascular complications exists for diurnal systemic hypertension. Peppard et al. (2000b), after controlling for known confounding risk factors for the development of hypertension (smoking, alcohol, weight, age, and sex), found a dose-response relationship between apnea and hypopnea and incident hypertension over a 4-year period (Figure 3–6).

Metabolic Complications

A number of investigators have identified metabolic dysregulation in OSAH. There is a dose-response relationship between the

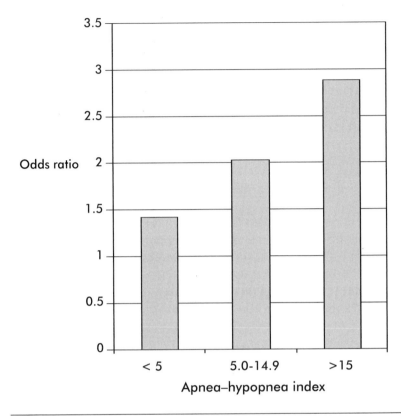

Figure 3–6. Obstructive sleep apnea/hypopnea: adjusted odds ratios for hypertension.

Adjusted odds ratio for incident hypertension, defined as blood pressure of at least 140/90 mm Hg or the use of antihypertensive medications for more than 8 years ($N=184$). Adjustments were made for baseline hypertension status, body habitus (body mass index, waist circumference, and neck circumference), weekly alcohol consumption, and cigarette use.

Source. Adapted from Peppard et al. 2000b.

AHI and biomarkers of the metabolic syndrome (serum glucose and insulin sensitivity), This relationship persists after controlling for concomitant obesity (Punjabi et al. 2003). Leptin, an adipokine that appears to play an important role in metabolic and ventilatory control, is elevated in OSAH (Ip et al. 2000). Leptin inhibits the synthesis of neuropeptide Y, a potent stimulator of food intake. Obese individuals typically have elevated circulating leptin levels, suggesting leptin resistance. The elevated leptin levels are not explained by obesity alone. Leptin levels in patients with OSAH are elevated compared with levels in matched obese control subjects, suggesting a direct effect of sleep-disordered breathing (Ip et al. 2000).

Neurocognitive Complications

One of the defining features of the OSAH syndrome is the symptom of daytime sleepiness. There is a dose-response relationship between the severity of sleep-disordered breathing and the complaint of daytime sleepiness (Gottlieb et al. 1999) (Figure 3–7). There is now strong evidence that the severity of OSAH also correlates with the risk of motor vehicle and occupational accidents. Terán-Santos et al. (1999) examined the risk of motor vehicle accidents, using a case-control design. After adjusting for a number of confounding variables, including body mass index, alcohol consumption, eyesight, medications, driving experience, and sleep schedule, the investigators found that subjects who had AHI >10 had a 7.2 odds ratio for having a traffic accident. Lindberg et al. (2001) prospectively evaluated the risk of occupational accidents in sleepy snorers over a 10-year period. In this community sample of more than 2,000 men, the risk for occupational accidents in sleepy snorers was 2.2 times that of the control population.

Neuropsychological performance in OSAH has been examined by a number of investigators. Beebe et al. (2003) performed a meta-analysis of the studies dealing with neuropsychological functioning in adults with untreated OSAH. The analysis involved 25 studies that met inclusion criteria, with a total of 1,092 patients and 899 control subjects. Untreated OSAH was associated with significant impact on vigilance, executive functioning, and coordination. There was negligible impact on intellectual and verbal functioning.

The association between depression and OSAH has been studied by a number of investigators, but the data linking OSAH to depression are conflicting (Sateia 2003). A recent analysis of a large managed care database examined the relationship between prescriptions for antidepressant and antihypertensive medications and a diagnosis of OSAH (Farney et al. 2004). The investi-

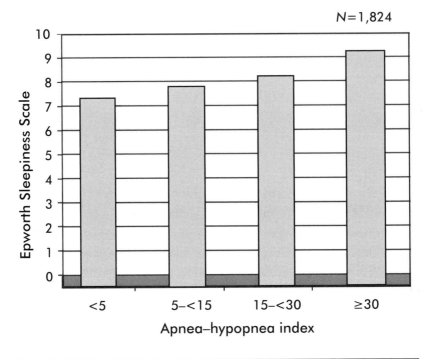

Figure 3–7. Obstructive sleep apnea/hypopnea: relationship of apnea-hypopnea index to sleepiness.

Relationship of self-reported daytime sleepiness (Epworth Sleepiness Scale score) to apnea-hypopnea index in a cross-sectional cohort (*N*=1,824).

Source. Adapted from Gottlieb et al. 1999.

gators identified a significant increase in the prevalence odds ratio for OSAH in patients prescribed either an antidepressant or an antihypertensive medication. The highest prevalence of OSAH was identified in young men and women (age 20–39 years) receiving both medications.

Sleepiness and impaired cognitive function undoubtedly affect quality of life. Large effect sizes have been reported for the impact of treatment of OSAH on quality of life as measured by both generic (Nottingham Health Profile [Hunt et al. 1985], SF-36 Health Survey [Ware and Sherbourne 1992]) and disease-specific quality of life measures (Engleman and Douglas 2004). In generic measures such as the SF-36, multiple domains are affected, including vitality and social function.

Controlled trials involving treatment of OSAH have demonstrated reversibility in measures of sleepiness, cognitive function, and quality of life (Engleman and Douglas 2004). These treatment data provide additional evidence for the biologic plausibility of the relationship of OSAH to neurocognitive impairment.

Diagnosis

A number of clinical clues increase the probability of diagnosing OSAH. Findings in the history and the physical exam can help the clinician select patients for physiological testing to confirm the diagnosis and assess its severity. Identifying patients at risk for OSAH is not difficult. The inability to diagnose OSAH is more commonly related to not considering the condition in the first place.

Clinical Presentation

The signs and symptoms of nightly loud snoring, breathing pauses during sleep, snorting, choking, or subjective daytime sleepiness all suggest the diagnosis of OSAH (Table 3–3). Obesity (particularly upper body obesity) and systemic hypertension may be present. In selected individuals, craniofacial abnormalities (retro or micrognathia) or soft tissue abnormalities, such as enlarged tonsils, lateral narrowing of the airway, or an elongated soft palate, may place the patient at risk for airway closure during sleep (Schellenberg et al. 2000; Zonato et al. 2003). Signs of right-sided heart failure in the absence of established heart disease may be associated with occult OSAH (Guidry et al. 2001).

Nocturnal hypoxemia associated with OSAH has been linked with modest pulmonary hypertension and peripheral edema due to right-sided heart failure. This clinical finding may be present in the absence of chronic obstructive pulmonary disease and appears to be related to the respiratory mechanical consequences associated with obesity (Bady et al. 2000). In patients without left ventricular dysfunction, Blankfield et al. (2000) reported a high prevalence of occult OSAH. Treatment of OSAH with continuous positive airway pressure is associated with improvement in pulmonary hypertension and right heart failure, suggesting a causal relationship (Sajkov et al. 2002).

Table 3–3.   Clinical presentation of obstructive sleep apnea/ hypopnea

History
    Nightly snoring
    Breathing pauses
    Snorting
    Choking
    Daytime sleepiness
    Menopause
    Nasal congestion
    Smoking
    Family history (genetics)

Physical exam finding
    Systemic hypertension
    Obesity (large neck)
    Nasal turbinate hypertrophy
    Long soft palate
    Lateral airway narrowing
    Tonsillar hypertrophy
    Retrognathia/micrognathia
    Right heart failure

Unfortunately, clinical findings alone do not provide sufficient precision to confirm a diagnosis of OSAH and stratify risk (Rowley et al. 2000; Schellenberg et al. 2000).

Laboratory Testing

Objective measurement and quantification of sleep and breathing in a sleep laboratory setting is currently the standard for confirming a diagnosis of OSAH in the United States. Sleep stages are identified in addition to the degree of sleep disruption that is due to sleep-disordered breathing events.

Sleep is analyzed by measuring electroencephalographic (via a central lead), bilateral electrooculographic, and submental electromyographic (chin) activity. Cardiopulmonary parameters are measured, including airflow, breathing effort, and oximetry and electrocardiogram readings. Sensors are applied to the legs to identify periodic leg movements that may be responsible for disrupting sleep. Recording of these measurements is illustrated in Figure 3–8.

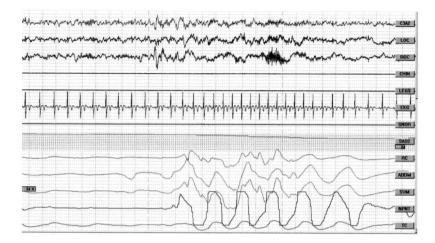

Figure 3–8. Polysomnogram epoch (30 seconds) showing an apnea with heart rate variability, electroencephalographic arousal, and oxyhemoglobin desaturation.

Note the lack of airflow in the nasal pressure (NPNT) and thermocouple (TC) signals associated with ongoing breathing effort in the rib cage (RC) and abdomen (ABDM) signals associated with oxyhemoglobin desaturation (SAO2), cortical arousal (C3A2) in conjunction with slowing and quickening of the heart rate (EKG).

Therapy

Relevant lifestyle interventions should be pursued in all patients. Positive pressure administered via a mask remains the initial treatment of choice. Second-line therapy can involve oral appliance therapy (OAP) and, in selected patients, upper airway surgery.

Lifestyle Interventions

Obesity is a major risk factor for OSAH. Weight loss has been demonstrated to improve both sleep and breathing (Peppard et al. 2000a). Avoiding sleep deprivation will not only decrease daytime sleepiness related to sleep debt, but also increase upper airway muscle tone. Alcohol and sedatives also negatively affect upper airway muscle tone. The magnitude of the impact of sedatives on the unstable upper airway is not well defined. If the patient clearly has positional OSAH, lateral position or head-of-bed elevation may be helpful.

Positive Pressure Therapy

Positive pressure delivered via nasal or nasal-oral mask reliably treats airway closure during sleep. It works primarily by "pneumatically splinting" the airway open during sleep (Figure 3–9), preferentially affecting the lateral pharyngeal wall. When a proper positive pressure prescription is performed, the treatment effect is virtually immediate.

Positive pressure can be applied as continuous positive airway pressure (CPAP) or as bilevel positive airway pressure (BPAP). With BPAP, the pressure setting is higher during inspiration than during expiration, taking advantage of the fact that during inspiration the airway pressure is more negative than during expiration. This is accomplished by the machine's sensing changes in airflow associated with breathing. Both CPAP and BPAP machines are electrically operated and are highly portable, usually weighing less than 10 pounds.

Of all the treatment options for OSAH, positive pressure therapy (primarily CPAP) has been most rigorously studied. Placebo-controlled, randomized clinical trials have documented a favorable effect on quality of life, objective daytime function, and blood pressure. CPAP improves insulin sensitivity, left ventricular function, pulmonary hypertension, endothelial function, cardiovascular mortality, and overall mortality (Blankfield et al. 2000; Harsch et al. 2002; Lavie 2003; Midelton et al. 2002; Peker et al. 2000; Punjabi et al. 2003; Resnick et al. 2003; Sajkov et al. 2002; Vgontzas et al. 2003).

Positive pressure therapy is unique in that unlike most medical treatments, it does not utilize drugs. Despite this striking difference, objective adherence to positive pressure therapy is similar to that for most medical regimens, at approximately 50% without structured educational interventions (Cramer 2003; Dekker et al. 1993).

Acceptance of and adherence to positive pressure can be improved with patient education and appropriate attention to patient–machine-related problems. In general, CPAP or BPAP is delivered via a nasal interface. Proper fit is essential. Nasal congestion and/or dryness needs to be treated. Patients with OSAH frequently report symptoms of nasal congestion prior to treatment. This problem can

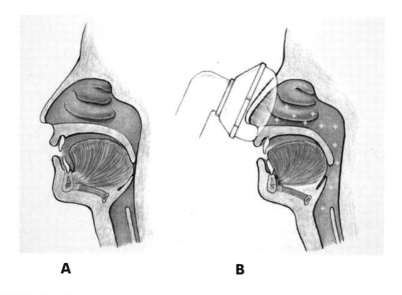

A   **B**

Figure 3–9.   Upper airway: without treatment (A) and with continuous positive airway pressure (CPAP) treatment (B).
Cross-sectional view of the upper airway illustrating closure at the level of the palate and base of tongue typically seen in obstructive sleep apnea **(A)** and **(B)** when the airway is pneumatically splinted open with continuous positive airway pressure.

be exacerbated by positive pressure therapy. The airflow through the nose at flow rates of 30–60 L/min (depending on the seal) can be drying to nasal mucosa. This frequently triggers rebound nasal congestion that precipitates mouth breathing. When the mouth opens, the machine increases the flow to maintain the set pressure, exacerbating the congestion. Heated humidifiers in line with the CPAP/BPAP unit can frequently improve the nasal dryness and subsequent congestion. Occasionally, a mask that covers both the nose and mouth can be helpful. In patients who are claustrophobic, desensitization may be helpful.

Oral Appliance Therapy

The goal of OAP is to modify the position of the mandible and the tongue to increase the upper airway size and favorably affect collapsibility. OAP should be regarded as second-line therapy for

OSAH because effective treatment requires multiple adjustments that require weeks to months to accomplish, treatment is not 100% effective, and objective adherence cannot be measured.

High-quality studies on the effectiveness of OAP are limited (Lim et al. 2003). Subjective sleepiness and sleep-disordered breathing are favorably affected in OAP patients compared with control subjects. A randomized, controlled trial has demonstrated a favorable effect on blood pressure (Gotsopoulos et al. 2004). Patients frequently prefer OAP to CPAP/BPAP. A patent (i.e., unobstructed) nasal airway is essential for optimal treatment.

Oral appliances for adults can be divided into two basic types: tongue-retaining devices (TRDs) and mandibular advancement devices (MADs) (Figure 3–10 and Figure 3–11). TRDs require suction applied to the anterior portion of the tongue to maintain tongue protrusion and an increase in the retrolingual airway. In addition, a degree of downward rotation of the mandible is achieved. TRDs can be used in edentulous patients. Many patients are bothered by the bulk of the TRD, and this negatively affects adherence.

MADs are the best-studied devices. Adjustable MADs are more comfortable and generally yield better results than nonadjustable "boil and bite" appliances. Sequential adjustment requires weeks to accomplish and thus limits the utility of MADs in severe OSAH that requires expeditious treatment. Patients with mild to moderate OSAH who do not accept positive pressure therapy are reasonable candidates for a trial of an oral appliance. Randomized, controlled trials have demonstrated that optimal therapy is achieved in approximately one-third of the subjects studied (Mehta et al. 2001). Case series data suggest that patients who respond best are those with mild OSAH, supine position–dependent OSAH, and snoring (Marklund et al. 2004).

It now clear that there are contraindications and complications associated with MAD treatment. Contraindications include an insufficient number of teeth to support the device, substantial tooth mobility, untreated periodontal disease, and active temporomandibular joint syndrome (Petit et al. 2002). At least 10 good teeth are required in each dental arch to adequately anchor the appliance. Side effects are usually mild and infrequently require intervention. Common side effects are mucosal dryness,

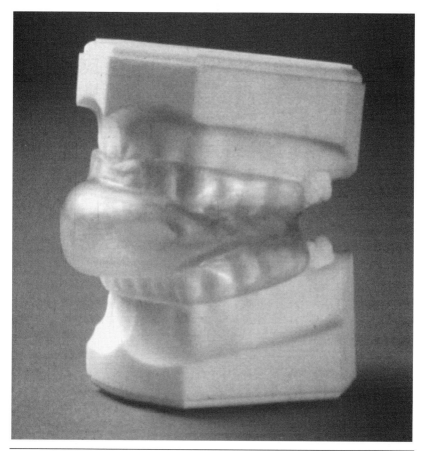

Figure 3–10. Tongue repositioning device (TRD).
Enlarges the airway by securing the tongue in an anterior position during sleep.

tooth discomfort, and hypersalivation (Fritsch et al. 2001). MADs are known to change occlusion over time. Regular dental follow-up is mandatory in patients using these devices long term.

Surgical Therapy

Surgical therapy has a small but definite role in the management of OSAH in adults. Surgery therapy can be broadly divided into two categories: 1) tracheostomy (bypass of the upper airway) and 2) reconstruction of the upper airway. Upper airway reconstruction can involve multiple sites from the nasopharynx to the epiglottis (see Figure 3–4).

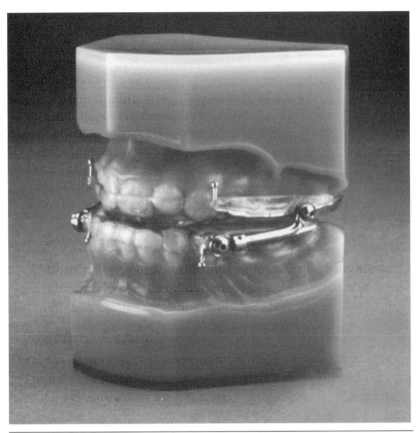

Figure 3–11. Mandibular advancement device (MAD).
Moves the mandible forward, enlarging the airway during sleep.

Tracheostomy was the original treatment for OSAH. CPAP or BPAP has largely replaced tracheostomy as the treatment of choice for severe OSAH. There remains a small group of patients with severe and potentially life-threatening OSAH who are intolerant of CPAP/BPAP and require tracheostomy.

Although the appearance of the tracheostomy can result in psychological and social morbidity, the treatment is well tolerated and results in cure of OSAH. Local complications involving the tracheal stoma can occur within the first year post tracheostomy (Thatcher and Maisel 2003). It is important to reassess the patient's nocturnal oxygen saturation after tracheostomy because the morbidly obese patient can still exhibit significant nonobstructive oxyhemoglobin desaturation in rapid eye movement sleep.

There is a lack of well-designed studies in the literature to definitively evaluate the effect of upper airway surgery on OSAH (Bridgman and Dunn 2000). A number of case series provide some support for surgery as a treatment option (Li et al. 2001, 2002; Riley et al. 2000).

The most commonly performed procedure is a uvulo-palatopharyngoplasty (UPP). The procedure involves altering the size and the stiffness of the soft palate. The UPP is highly effective in treating loud snoring. The impact on OSAH is less certain, with success ranging from 7% to 60% (McGuirt et al. 1995; Sher 1995). Three types of palatal surgery that involve different surgical approaches have been described. The traditional approach involves trimming the palate with a scalpel and usually performing a concomitant tonsillectomy (Figure 3–12). This is performed in the operating room under general anesthesia. A UPP can also be performed by using a laser to cut the palatal tissue. The benefit of this approach is that the procedure can be performed under local anesthesia and titrated to effect (elimination of snoring) in the outpatient clinic (Finkelstein et al. 2002; Littner et al. 2001). The third type of palatal procedure involves using a needle to deliver radiofrequency energy (usually about 400 joules) to "stiffen" the palate. The advantage is significantly less pain because of the lack of a mucosal wound. The detriment is that the long-term effect is not as robust or sustaining as that achieved by cutting the palatal tissue with a scalpel or laser (Blumen et al. 2002).

Reconstruction of the upper airway is a better option than tracheostomy from a cosmetic perspective but unfortunately is associated with less certain results. It is now clear that in OSAH airway closure occurs at more than one site during sleep (Morrison et al. 1993). In order to effectively treat OSAH, airway closure involving the palate and base of tongue must be considered. A phased approach to upper airway reconstruction has been popularized by the Stanford group (Riley et al. 1993). Phase I surgery generally involves a palatoplasty and a genioglossal advancement procedure. Phase II surgery involves maxillomandibular advancement (Figure 3–13). Phase I surgery is associated with low morbidity but less than optimal results, with reported suc-

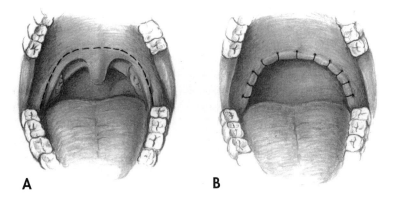

Figure 3–12. Uvulopalatopharyngoplasty (UPP) preoperative and postoperative views.
A: Appearance of the oropharynx prior to UPP, with dotted line identifying site of incision. **B:** Postoperatively, with sutures in place.

cess rates ranging from 22% to 60% (Bettega et al. 2000; Riley et al. 1993). Phase II surgery is more effective, with reported success rates ranging from 75% to 100%. Phase II procedures, although less painful overall, are associated with transient trauma and possible damage to the inferior alveolar nerve. These procedures produce changes in occlusion that invariably require postoperative orthodontics.

Upper airway reconstruction for OSAH is an elective surgery that should be contemplated only after positive pressure techniques (CPAP/BPAP) have been tried. If there are cosmetic considerations such as retrognathia or micrognathia, particularly in a young adult, this treatment may make good sense. PSG should be performed postoperatively to objectively measure improvement in the AHI and sleep quality, regardless of the impact on snoring.

Relevance to Psychiatric Practice

The most common neurocognitive symptoms associated with OSAH are fatigue and daytime sleepiness. Fatigue and daytime sleepiness can be misinterpreted as depression. If OSAH is not considered as a possible diagnosis, the patient may be ineffec-

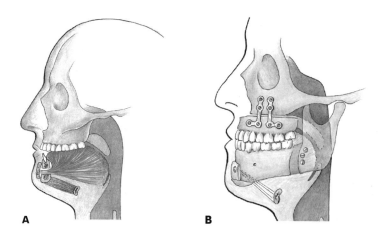

Figure 3–13. Cross-sectional view of the upper airway illustrating surgical changes.
A: Phase 1, uvulopalatopharyngoplasty (UPP) and genioglossal advancement.
B: Phase 2, maxillomandibular advancement.

tively treated. On the other hand, fatigue that persists after adequate treatment for OSAH has been established may indicate concomitant untreated depression (Bardwell et al. 2003) or possibly residual daytime sleepiness related to OSAH. Bardwell et al. (2003) explored this relationship in untreated OSAH patients. After controlling for apnea severity, the authors found that the complaint of fatigue, as measured by the fatigue-inertia subscale of the Profile of Mood States, had a significant effect on the score for the symptom of depression. Given the high prevalence of both depressive disorders and OSAH in the population, true co-occurrence of these conditions is expected to be fairly common.

Once depression and chronic sleep deprivation are excluded, residual daytime sleepiness may be related to OSAH (Pack et al. 2001). Investigators using magnetic resonance imaging have reported gray matter loss in the frontal and parietal cortex, temporal lobe, anterior cingulate, hippocampus, and cerebellum in OSAH patients (Macey et al. 2002; Morrell et al. 2003). Veasey et al. (2004a), studying mice exposed to long-term intermittent hypoxia (biologically similar to OSAH), found significant oxidative injuries in the wake-promoting regions of the basal forebrain and brainstem. These investigators also found that compared with controls, these mice had decreased sleep latencies measured with a murine multiple sleep latency test (Veasey et al. 2004b).

Modafinil is a novel wake-promoting drug whose mechanism of action has not been completely characterized. It appears to work at least in part on the dopamine system in promoting wakefulness (Saper and Scammell 2004). The drug has been shown to be effective as an adjunctive therapy for OSAH patients who experience unacceptable symptoms of daytime sleepiness despite adequate treatment with positive pressure therapy (Pack et al. 2001).

Insomnia can also be encountered in the OSAH patient. The true prevalence of insomnia in patients with OSAH is unknown. Krakow et al. (2001) reported problematic insomnia in 50% of a retrospective cohort of patients with OSAH. There are no data specifically addressing the impact of insomnia on the ability to accept and adhere to CPAP/BPAP therapy. It is biologically plausible that concomitant insomnia may affect treatment of OSAH. The degree of subjective sleepiness as measured by the Epworth Sleepiness Scale (ESS) has been shown to affect treatment. In a consecutive case series of 1,211 patients, McArdle et al. (1999) reported that an ESS score >10 predicted long-term adherence to CPAP.

Summary

Obstructive sleep apnea is a common clinical condition that is associated with significant metabolic, cardiovascular, and neurocognitive morbidity and mortality. Clinical clues such as heavy snoring, observed apnea, and daytime sleepiness suggest the diagnosis. The diagnosis must be confirmed by an overnight sleep study. The initial medical therapy of choice is nasal CPAP. Treatment with nasal CPAP is highly effective in patients with moderate to severe OSA and daytime sleepiness. The evidence clearly demonstrates that in addition to eliminating snoring, this technique substantially improves nocturnal cardiovascular function, daytime sleepiness, and quality of life. The current literature supports the notion that long-term treatment may favorably affect cardiovascular outcomes. Selected patients who do not accept or adhere to nasal CPAP may benefit from OAP therapy or surgery.

Mental health consultants frequently encounter patients with complaints of poor quality of sleep and daytime sleepiness. Identification and proper treatment of OSAH can diminish daytime sleepiness, improve quality of life, and have a favorable effect on cardiovascular comorbidities. Identifying and treating insomnia in OSAH patients may favorably affect adherence to positive pressure treatment as well as improve quality of life.

References

American Academy of Sleep Medicine: Sleep-related breathing disorders in adults: recommendations for syndrome definition and measurement techniques in clinical research. The report of an American Academy of Sleep Medicine Task Force. Sleep 22:667–689, 1999

Ancoli-Israel S, Klauber MR, Stepnowsky C, et al: Sleep-disordered breathing in African-American elderly. Am J Respir Crit Care Med 152:1946–1949, 1995

Bady E, Achkar A, Pascal S, et al: Pulmonary arterial hypertension in patients with sleep apnoea syndrome. Thorax 55:934–939, 2000

Bardwell WA, Moore P, Ancoli-Israel S, et al: Fatigue in obstructive sleep apnea: driven by depressive symptoms instead of apnea severity? Am J Psychiatry 160:350–355, 2003

Beebe DW, Groesz L, Wells C, et al: The neuropsychological effects of obstructive sleep apnea: a meta-analysis of norm-referenced and case-controlled data. Sleep 26:298–307, 2003

Bettega G, Pepin JL, Veale D, et al: Obstructive sleep apnea syndrome: fifty-one consecutive patients treated by maxillofacial surgery. Am J Respir Crit Care Med 162:641–649, 2000

Bixler EO, Vgontzas AN, Lin HM, et al: Prevalence of sleep-disordered breathing in women: effects of gender. Am J Respir Crit Care Med 163:608–613, 2001

Blankfield RP, Hudgel DW, Tapolyai AA, et al: Bilateral leg edema, obesity, pulmonary hypertension, and obstructive sleep apnea. Arch Intern Med 160:2357–2362 [erratum, 160:2650], 2000

Blumen MB, Dahan S, Fleury B, et al: Radiofrequency ablation for the treatment of mild to moderate obstructive sleep apnea. Laryngoscope 112:2086–2092, 2002

Bridgman SA, Dunn KM: Surgery for obstructive sleep apnoea. Cochrane Database Syst Rev (2):CD001004, 2000

Cramer J: Medicine partnerships. Heart 89 (suppl 2):19–21, 2003

Dekker FW, Dieleman FE, Kaptein AA, et al: Compliance with pulmonary medication in general practice. Eur Respir J 6:886–890, 1993

Engleman HM, Douglas NJ: Sleep, 4: sleepiness, cognitive function, and quality of life in obstructive sleep apnoea/hypopnoea syndrome. Thorax 59:618–622, 2004

Farney RJ, Lugo A, Jensen RL, et al: Simultaneous use of antidepressant and antihypertensive medications increases likelihood of diagnosis of obstructive sleep apnea syndrome. Chest 125:1279–1285, 2004

Finkelstein Y, Stein G, Ophir D, et al: Laser-assisted uvulopalatoplasty for the management of obstructive sleep apnea: myths and facts. Arch Otolaryngol Head Neck Surg 128:429–434, 2002

Fritsch KM, Iseli A, Russi EW, et al: Side effects of mandibular advancement devices for sleep apnea treatment. Am J Respir Crit Care Med 164:813–818, 2001

Gleeson K, Zwillich CW, White DP: The influence of increasing ventilatory effort on arousal from sleep. Am Rev Respir Dis 142:295–300, 1990

Gotsopoulos H, Kelly JJ, Cistulli PA: Oral appliance therapy reduces blood pressure in obstructive sleep apnea: a randomized, controlled trial. Sleep 27:934–941, 2004

Gottlieb DJ, Whitney CW, Bonekat WH, et al: Relation of sleepiness to respiratory disturbance index: the Sleep Heart Health Study. Am J Respir Crit Care Med 159:502–507, 1999

Guidry UC, Mendes LA, Evans JC, et al: Echocardiographic features of the right heart in sleep-disordered breathing: the Framingham Heart Study. Am J Respir Crit Care Med 164:933–938, 2001

Harsch IA, Schahin SP, Fuchs FS, et al: Insulin resistance, hyperleptinemia, and obstructive sleep apnea in Launois-Bensaude syndrome. Obes Res 10:625–632, 2002

Ip MS, Lam KS, Ho C, et al: Serum leptin and vascular risk factors in obstructive sleep apnea. Chest 118:580–586, 2000

Krakow B, Melendrez D, Ferreira E, et al: Prevalence of insomnia symptoms in patients with sleep-disordered breathing. Chest 120:1923–1929, 2001

Lavie L: Obstructive sleep apnoea syndrome—an oxidative stress disorder. Sleep Med Rev 7:35–51, 2003

Li KK, Riley RW, Powell NB, et al: Obstructive sleep apnea surgery: genioglossus advancement revisited. J Oral Maxillofac Surg 59:1181–1184, 2001

Li KK, Powell NB, Riley RW, et al: Distraction osteogenesis in adult obstructive sleep apnea surgery: a preliminary report. J Oral Maxillofac Surg 60:6–10, 2002

Lim J, Lasserson TJ, Fleetham J, et al: Oral appliances for obstructive sleep apnoea. Cochrane Database Syst Rev (4):CD004435, 2003

Lindberg E, Carter N, Gislason T, et al: Role of snoring and daytime sleepiness in occupational accidents. Am J Respir Crit Care Med 164:2031–2035, 2001

Littner M, Kushida CA, Hartse K, et al: Practice parameters for the use of laser-assisted uvulopalatoplasty: an update for 2000. Sleep 24:603–619, 2001

Macey PM, Henderson LA, Macey KE, et al: Brain morphology associated with obstructive sleep apnea. Am J Respir Crit Care Med 166:1382–1387, 2002

Marklund M, Stenlund H, Franklin KA: Mandibular advancement devices in 630 men and women with obstructive sleep apnea and snoring: tolerability and predictors of treatment success. Chest 125:1270–1278, 2004

McArdle N, Devereux G, Heidarnejad H, et al: Long-term use of CPAP therapy for sleep apnea/hypopnea syndrome. Am J Respir Crit Care Med 159:1108–1114, 1999

McGuirt WF Jr, Johnson JT, Sanders MH: Previous tonsillectomy as prognostic indicator for success of uvulopalatopharyngoplasty. Laryngoscope 105:1253–1255, 1995

Hunt SM, McEwen J, McKenna SP: Measuring health status: a new tool for clinicians and epidemiologists. J R Coll Gen Pract 35:185–188, 1985

Mehta A, Qian J, Petocz P, et al: A randomized, controlled study of a mandibular advancement splint for obstructive sleep apnea. Am J Respir Crit Care Med 163:1457–1461, 2001

Midelton GT, Frishman WH, Passo SS: Congestive heart failure and continuous positive airway pressure therapy: support of a new modality for improving the prognosis and survival of patients with advanced congestive heart failure. Heart Dis 4:102–109, 2002

Morrell MJ, McRobbie DW, Quest RA, et al: Changes in brain morphology associated with obstructive sleep apnea. Sleep Med 4:451–454, 2003

Morrison DL, Launois SH, Isono S, et al: Pharyngeal narrowing and closing pressures in patients with obstructive sleep apnea. Am Rev Respir Dis 148:606–611, 1993

Pack AI, Black JE, Schwartz JR, et al: Modafinil as adjunct therapy for daytime sleepiness in obstructive sleep apnea. Am J Respir Crit Care Med 164:1675–1681, 2001

Peker Y, Hedner J, Kraiczi H, et al: Respiratory disturbance index: an independent predictor of mortality in coronary artery disease. Am J Respir Crit Care Med 162:81–86, 2000

Peppard PE, Young T, Palta M, et al: Longitudinal study of moderate weight change and sleep-disordered breathing. JAMA 284:3015–3021, 2000a

Peppard PE, Young T, Palta M, et al: Prospective study of the association between sleep-disordered breathing and hypertension. N Engl J Med 342:1378–1384, 2000b

Petit FX, Pepin JL, Bettega G, et al: Mandibular advancement devices: rate of contraindications in 100 consecutive obstructive sleep apnea patients. Am J Respir Crit Care Med 166:274–278, 2002

Punjabi NM, Ahmed MM, Polotsky VY, et al: Sleep-disordered breathing, glucose intolerance, and insulin resistance. Rev Respir Physiol Neurobiol 136:167–178, 2003

Resnick HE, Redline S, Shahar E, et al: Diabetes and sleep disturbances: findings from the Sleep Heart Health Study. Diabetes Care 26:702–709, 2003

Riley RW, Powell NB, Guilleminault C: Obstructive sleep apnea syndrome: a review of 306 consecutively treated surgical patients. Otolaryngol Head Neck Surg 108:117–125, 1993

Riley RW, Powell NB, Li KK, et al: Surgery and obstructive sleep apnea: long-term clinical outcomes. Otolaryngol Head Neck Surg 122:415–421, 2000

Rowley JA, Aboussouan LS, Badr MS: The use of clinical prediction formulas in the evaluation of obstructive sleep apnea. Sleep 23:929–938, 2000

Sajkov D, Wang T, Saunders NA, et al: Continuous positive airway pressure treatment improves pulmonary hemodynamics in patients with obstructive sleep apnea. Am J Respir Crit Care Med 165:152–158, 2002

Saper CB, Scammell TE: Modafinil: a drug in search of a mechanism. Sleep 27:11–12, 2004

Sateia MJ: Neuropsychological impairment and quality of life in obstructive sleep apnea. Clin Chest Med 24:249–259, 2003

Schellenberg JB, Maislin G, Schwab RJ: Physical findings and the risk for obstructive sleep apnea: the importance of oropharyngeal structures. Am J Respir Crit Care Med 162:740–748, 2000

Shahar E, Whitney CW, Redline S, et al: Sleep-disordered breathing and cardiovascular disease: cross-sectional results of the Sleep Heart Health Study. Am J Respir Crit Care Med 163:19–25, 2001

Sher AE: Update on upper airway surgery for obstructive sleep apnea. Curr Opin Pulm Med 1:504–511, 1995

Somers VK, Dyken ME, Clary MP, et al: Sympathetic neural mechanisms in obstructive sleep apnea. J Clin Invest 96:1897–1904, 1995

Strollo PJ Jr, Rogers RM: Obstructive sleep apnea. N Engl J Med 334:99–104, 1996

Terán-Santos J, Jimenez-Gomez A, Cordero-Guevara J: The association between sleep apnea and the risk of traffic accidents. Cooperative Group Burgos-Santander. N Engl J Med 340:847–851, 1999

Thatcher GW, Maisel RH: The long-term evaluation of tracheostomy in the management of severe obstructive sleep apnea. Laryngoscope 113:201–204, 2003

Tishler PV, Larkin EK, Schluchter MD, et al: Incidence of sleep-disordered breathing in an urban adult population: the relative importance of risk factors in the development of sleep-disordered breathing. JAMA 289:2230–2237, 2003

Tsai WH, Flemons WW, Whitelaw WA, et al: A comparison of apnea-hypopnea indices derived from different definitions of hypopnea. Am J Respir Crit Care Med 159:43–48, 1999

Veasey SC, Davis CW, Fenik P, et al: Long-term intermittent hypoxia in mice: protracted hypersomnolence with oxidative injury to sleep-wake brain regions. Sleep 27:194–201, 2004a

Veasey SC, Yeou-Jey H, Thayer P, et al: Murine Multiple Sleep Latency Test: phenotyping sleep propensity in mice. Sleep 27:388–393, 2004b

Vgontzas AN, Bixler EO, Chrousos GP: Metabolic disturbances in obesity versus sleep apnoea: the importance of visceral obesity and insulin resistance. J Intern Med 254:32–44, 2003

Ware JE Jr, Sherbourne CD: The MOS 36-item short-form health survey (SF-36), I: conceptual framework and item selection. Med Care 30:473–483, 1992

Young T, Palta M, Dempsey J, et al: The occurrence of sleep-disordered breathing among middle-aged adults. N Engl J Med 328:1230–1235, 1993

Young T, Peppard PE, Gottlieb DJ: Epidemiology of obstructive sleep apnea: a population health perspective. Am J Respir Crit Care Med 165:1217–1239, 2002a

Young T, Shahar E, Nieto FJ, et al: Predictors of sleep-disordered breathing in community-dwelling adults: the Sleep Heart Health Study. Arch Intern Med 162:893–900, 2002b

Zonato AI, Bittencourt LR, Martinho FL, et al: Association of systematic head and neck physical examination with severity of obstructive sleep apnea-hypopnea syndrome. Laryngoscope 113:973–980, 2003

Chapter 4

Narcolepsy and Syndromes of Central Nervous System–Mediated Sleepiness

Jed E. Black, M.D.
Seiji Nishino, M.D., Ph.D.
Stephen N. Brooks, M.D.

The complaints of tiredness, fatigue, sedation, and sleepiness are common among patients with psychiatric disorders. Many factors contribute to the experience of diminished alertness across individuals with such complaints. Potential contributing elements include presumed physiological epiphenomena of primary pathological conditions (e.g., "hypersomnia" in "atypical" depression), medication effects, use or abuse of sedating substances, sleep disruption, advanced or delayed circadian rhythm phase, voluntary or involuntary sleep restriction, and other sleep disorders (e.g., obstructive sleep apnea syndrome). The careful characterization of the complaint is of key importance in the evaluation of suboptimal alertness or fatigue for appropriate diagnosis and symptom management—primary treatment, when possible, or secondary amelioration.

Occasionally, patients will manifest somnolence or frank sleepiness—unrelated to factors such as those noted above or to the primary psychiatric condition they have—as a result of distinct central nervous system (CNS) dysfunction. Sometimes the CNS condition of excessive sleepiness is comorbid with a primary psychiatric disorder. However, not infrequently, the patient receives the diagnosis of a psychiatric illness when none is present. Comorbid disorders of somnolence or excessive daytime sleepiness (EDS) add frustration to the diagnostic workup and complexity to the treatment of individuals with psychiatric disorders. Sleep-related conditions that arise from CNS dysfunction tend to be less familiar to the clinician. Indeed, lack of an understanding of these conditions not only leads to their being misdiagnosed or overlooked, but at times results in gross mismanagement (e.g., the use of antipsychotic medications for narcolepsy-related hypnagogic hallucinations).

Narcolepsy is the most well known and extensively studied of the EDS conditions arising from CNS dysfunction, yet it, too, is often misunderstood and misdiagnosed. Idiopathic hypersomnia, the recurrent hypersomnias, and EDS associated with nervous system disorders also must be understood in order to provide appropriate evaluation and management. In this chapter, we summarize the distinguishing features of these clinical syndromes of primary EDS and provide a brief overview of their pharmacologic management. Additionally, we review the great advances in our understanding of the pathophysiology of narcolepsy that have occurred in the past few years.

Epidemiology of Excessive Daytime Sleepiness

The epidemiology of EDS has been explored, using a variety of research methods, in many countries around the world. The largest and most comprehensive representative population survey was performed across four Western European countries (the United Kingdom, Germany, Spain, and Italy). Substantial EDS, defined as meeting three parameters of marked sleepiness during three or more days a week, was reported in 15% of this combined population (Ohayon et al. 2002). Smaller population surveys in the United States have been conducted. Two recent polls suggest that 15%–16% of the U.S. population may experience EDS that interferes with daily activities a few days a week or more (National Sleep Foundation 2002, 2003). These data do not indicate the percentage of sleepy individuals whose sleepiness results from insufficient sleep or environmental factors rather than from pathological causes of EDS.

The prevalence of syndromes of CNS-mediated sleepiness is much more difficult to assess than that of EDS in the general population and, with the exception of narcolepsy, it remains poorly characterized. Data gathered in U.S. and Western European narcolepsy studies demonstrate a fairly consistent prevalence of approximately 0.05%, although rates as low as 0.002% and as high as 0.16% have been reported for Israel and Japan, respectively (Mignot 1998). In general, the published literature on the epidemiology of CNS-mediated EDS syndromes indicates a total prevalence that ranges from as high as 2%–3% to much less than 1% of the population.

Insufficient Sleep and Primary Syndromes of Excessive Daytime Sleepiness

Fragmented Sleep and Insufficient Sleep

Essential in the evaluation of patients presenting with EDS is the determination of the presence or absence of the two most common causes of EDS: 1) fragmented sleep due to extrinsic or intrinsic factors and 2) insufficient sleep. Fragmented sleep, predominantly microfragmentation resulting from such conditions as sleep-related breathing disorders (e.g., obstructive sleep apnea syndrome) and periodic limb movement disorder (PLMD), is an important consideration in the evaluation of EDS. These conditions are addressed in Chapter 3, "Sleep Apnea," and Chapter 5, "Restless Legs Syndrome," in this volume. The most common cause of daytime sleepiness is insufficient sleep, which may reflect poor sleep "hygiene" (behaviors negatively affecting sleep) or self-imposed or socially dictated sleep deprivation. Insufficient sleep is expected to lead to frank EDS, yet the more common subjective complaints are those of tiredness, lack of energy, or fatigue. Additionally, decrements in attention, learning capacity, short-term memory, and psychomotor performance, with or without EDS, may be present. Moreover, irritability, poor impulse control, or other forms of mood instability may exist alone or in concert with the above-noted features in individuals with insufficient sleep.

Primary Disorders of Excessive Daytime Sleepiness

Two diagnostic classification manuals are commonly used to specify diagnostic criteria for disorders of primary EDS. DSM-IV-TR (American Psychiatric Association 2000) subcategorizes these disorders into *narcolepsy* and *primary hypersomnia*; the latter includes all non-narcolepsy forms of primary EDS. The *International Classification of Sleep Disorders* (ICSD; American Sleep Disorders Association 1997) subcategorizes primary EDS into narcolepsy, idiopathic hypersomnia, recurrent hypersomnia, and posttraumatic hypersomnia. We have selected the ICSD format to organize this review, but we suggest the expansion of the posttraumatic category to include CNS pathology in addition to trauma.

As suggested by both DSM-IV-TR and ICSD, several entities may be regarded as primary disorders of EDS. Narcolepsy, the best known and the most completely understood disorder of this group, will be considered at greater length; other clinical syndromes will be reviewed more briefly. Patients with these CNS-mediated EDS syndromes commonly receive a misdiagnosis of a mood disorder and are treated with antidepressant therapy.

Narcolepsy

Narcolepsy is a syndrome of unknown etiology characterized by a profound degree of EDS. Narcolepsy usually occurs in association with cataplexy and other symptoms and signs, including hypnagogic or hypnopompic hallucinations, sleep paralysis, automatic behavior, and disrupted nocturnal sleep (American Sleep Disorders Association 1997). Symptoms most often begin during adolescence or young adulthood. However, narcolepsy may also occur earlier in childhood or not until the third or fourth decade of life. The impact of narcolepsy on quality of life is equal to that of other chronic neurologic disorders, such as Parkinson's disease (Beusterien et al. 1999). No symptom or sign of narcolepsy is specific to narcolepsy; even cataplexy unrelated to narcolepsy occurs, rarely, either as an isolated symptom or in conjunction with other conditions. Unfortunately, the average duration from symptom onset to the conferring of an accurate diagnosis is greater than 10 years. This substantial delay in diagnosis is largely due to clinicians' lack of education about and experience with this disorder.

Symptoms of narcolepsy include the following:

- *Sleepiness or excessive daytime sleepiness.* The EDS of narcolepsy presents as an increased propensity to fall asleep, nod, or doze easily in relaxed or sedentary situations, or a need to exert extra effort to avoid sleeping in these situations. Additionally, irresistible or overwhelming urges to sleep commonly occur from time to time during wakeful periods in untreated patients. These "sleep attacks" are not instantaneous lapses into sleep, as is often thought by the general public, but represent episodes of profound sleepiness similar to that caused by severe sleep deprivation or other severe sleep disorders. Many but not all patients with narcolepsy find that brief naps and longer sleep periods can be temporarily restorative or refreshing. This contrasts with the response to naps or sleep observed in idiopathic hypersomnia, wherein sleep of any duration is rarely restorative. In addition to frank sleepiness, the excessive daytime sleepiness of narcolepsy can cause or contribute to related symptoms, including poor memory, reduced concentration or attention, and irritability.

- *Cataplexy.* Cataplexy is the partial or complete loss of bilateral voluntary muscle tone in response to strong emotion. The reduced muscle tone may be minimal, occur in a few muscle groups, and cause minimal symptoms such as bilateral ptosis, head drooping, slurred speech, or dropping things from the hand. On the other hand, it may be so severe that total body paralysis occurs, resulting in complete collapse. Cataplectic events usually last from a few seconds to 2 or 3 minutes, but they occasionally continue longer (Honda 1988). The patient is usually alert and oriented during the event despite the inability to respond; thus, cataplectic episodes are distinct from sleep episodes. Positive emotions such as laughter trigger cataplexy more commonly than negative emotions. However, any strong emotion is a potential trigger (Gelb et al. 1994). Startling stimuli, stress, physical fatigue, and sleepiness may also be important triggers or factors that exacerbate cataplexy.

According to epidemiologic studies, cataplexy is found in 60%–100% of patients with narcolepsy. The onset of cataplexy is most frequently simultaneous with or within a few months of the onset of EDS, but in some cases cataplexy may not develop until many years after initial onset of EDS (Honda 1988).

- *Hypnagogic or hypnopompic hallucinations.* These phenomena are visual (most common), tactile, auditory, or multisensory events, usually brief but occasionally continuing for a few minutes, that occur at the transition from wakefulness to sleep (hypnagogic) or from sleep to wakefulness (hypnopompic). Hallucinations may contain elements of dream sleep and consciousness combined, and they are often bizarre or disturbing to patients. Occasionally, patients who experience these episodes are misdiagnosed with a psychotic syndrome and inappropriately treated with antipsychotic medications.
- *Sleep paralysis.* Sleep paralysis is the inability to move, lasting from a few seconds to minutes, during the transition from sleep to wakefulness or from wakefulness to sleep. Episodes of sleep paralysis may alarm patients, particularly those who experience the sensation of being unable to breathe. Although accessory respiratory muscles may not be active during these episodes, diaphragmatic activity continues and air exchange remains adequate.
- *Other symptoms.* Other commonly reported symptoms in narcolepsy include *automatic behavior*—absent-minded behavior or speech that is often nonsensical and that the patient does not remember because of extreme sleepiness. In addition, many individuals with narcolepsy report *fragmented nocturnal sleep*— that is, frequent awakenings during the night.

Hypnagogic hallucinations, sleep paralysis, and automatic behavior are not specific to narcolepsy and may occur in other sleep disorders, as well as in healthy individuals. These symptoms are, however, far more common and occur with much greater frequency in narcolepsy.

The following tools are available for the evaluation of narcolepsy:

- *Polysomnography.* Nocturnal polysomnography (PSG) is not essential in the diagnostic workup when straightforward cataplexy accompanies EDS. However, it remains an important part of the evaluation process, primarily to exclude other conditions that occur in narcolepsy at a higher than normal rate, such as obstructive sleep apnea (see Chapter 3, "Sleep Apnea"), PLMD (see Chapter 5, "Restless Legs Syndrome"), and rapid eye movement (REM) sleep behavior disorder. These conditions may contribute to the sleepiness or nocturnal sleep disruption the patient may be experiencing (Overeem et al. 2001). Additionally, individuals with narcolepsy may demonstrate sleep-onset REM periods during nocturnal PSG. Normally, nocturnal sleep begins with a long period of non–rapid eye movement (NREM) sleep (see Chapter 1, "Introduction").
- *Daytime sleep studies.* Daytime nap studies, in the form of the multiple sleep latency test (MSLT), usually demonstrate substantially reduced sleep latency coupled with sleep-onset REM periods (SOREMPs) in patients with narcolepsy. This test subjects the patient to four or five 20-minute nap opportunities, under PSG monitoring, at 2-hour intervals across the morning and afternoon. During testing, the patient is in bed in a dark room and is instructed to try to fall asleep. Average MSLT sleep latencies for *normal control subjects* are 12–15 minutes, but latencies for patients with narcolepsy with cataplexy average approximately 2–4 minutes (US Xyrem in Narcolepsy Multi-center Study Group 2002); however, there can be substantial variability across patients and within patients. SOREMPs are not specific for narcolepsy, but the occurrence of two or more of these events during the MSLT, in the setting of objective marked sleepiness and without another explanation for their occurrence (e.g., sleep deprivation, REM-suppressant medication rebound, altered sleep schedule, obstructive sleep apnea, or delayed sleep phase syndrome), is suggestive of narcolepsy. The presence of two or more SOREMPs can be found in a subset of patients with any of the other conditions just mentioned. These conditions are far more prevalent than narcolepsy. Therefore, the specificity for narcolepsy of two or more SOREMPs on the MSLT is low, but most patients with straightforward narcolepsy will manifest this finding.

- *Cerebrospinal fluid (CSF) hypocretin assessment.* As discussed below in the section on the pathophysiology of narcolepsy, many, but not all, patients with narcolepsy have very low or undetectable levels of the peptide neurotransmitter hypocretin in the CSF (Nishino et al. 2000b; Mignot et al. 2002). Such low levels of CSF hypocretin are not specific for narcolepsy. However, when used to assess patients for narcolepsy, low CSF hypocretin appears to be a much more specific test than the MSLT. Whether this test is more sensitive than the MSLT has yet to be determined.

- *Histocompatibility human leukocyte antigen (HLA) testing.* A very strong but incomplete correlation exists between narcolepsy (with cataplexy) and the HLA subtype DQB1* 0602. However, this subtype is also very common in the general population (occurring in about 20% in the United States) and is not at all specific nor sensitive for narcolepsy (Mignot 1998). HLA testing is therefore not useful in confirming or excluding the diagnosis of narcolepsy, and in fact may lead a clinician to inappropriate diagnostic conclusions.

Idiopathic Hypersomnia

Idiopathic hypersomnia (previously labeled *idiopathic CNS hypersomnia*) is an incompletely defined disorder characterized by EDS. This diagnosis has been used as a nosologic haven for classifying individuals with excessive somnolence but without the classic features of narcolepsy or another disorder known to cause EDS, such as sleep apnea. Without doubt, many patients have received diagnoses of idiopathic hypersomnia who actually had other disorders, such as narcolepsy without cataplexy, delayed sleep phase syndrome, or upper airway resistance syndrome, a subtle variant of the obstructive sleep apnea syndrome (Guilleminault et al. 1993). Roth (1976) described monosymptomatic and polysymptomatic forms of idiopathic hypersomnia, the former characterized by EDS alone and the latter characterized by EDS, prolonged nocturnal sleep time, and marked difficulty with awakening. Others have suggested that the category of idiopathic hypersomnia is heterogeneous, including individuals with EDS with or without one or more of the other features of Roth's polysymptomatic form (Aldrich 1996).

Idiopathic hypersomnia is believed to be less common than narcolepsy; estimation of prevalence, however, is elusive because strict diagnostic criteria are lacking and no specific biological marker has been identified. Typically, onset of symptoms occurs in adolescence or early adulthood. Symptoms generally persist for life, although a few patients with idiopathic hypersomnia have improved over time or attained complete remission of symptoms (Bassetti and Aldrich 1997; Billiard and Dauvilliers 2001; Bruck and Parkes 1996). The etiology of the disorder is not known, but viral illnesses, including Guillain-Barré syndrome, hepatitis, mononucleosis, and atypical viral pneumonia, may herald the onset of sleepiness in a subset of patients. EDS may occur as part of the acute illness, but it persists after the other symptoms subside. Familial cases are known to occur, with increased frequency of HLA-Cw2 and HLA-DR11 (Montplaisir and Poirier 1988). Some of these patients have associated symptoms suggesting autonomic nervous system dysfunction, including orthostatic hypotension, syncope, vascular headaches, and peripheral vascular complaints. Most patients with idiopathic hypersomnia have neither a family history nor an obvious associated viral illness. Little is known about the pathophysiology of idiopathic hypersomnia. No animal model is available for study. Neurochemical studies examining CSF have suggested that patients with idiopathic hypersomnia may have altered noradrenergic system function (Faull et al. 1983, 1986; Montplaisir et al. 1982).

The clinical picture of idiopathic hypersomnia varies among individual patients. The disorder may be mistaken for narcolepsy if a careful history is not taken. The two disorders share several common features, including similar age of onset, lifelong persistence after onset, EDS as the primary symptom, and familial clustering of some cases. However, essential differences between the disorders become apparent in the history and in diagnostic studies (see Table 4–1). Patients with idiopathic CNS hypersomnia present with EDS, but with neither cataplexy (although some patients have episodes of sleep paralysis or hypnagogic hallucinations) nor significant nocturnal sleep disruption (Billiard and Dauvilliers 2001). They complain of daytime sleepiness that interferes with normal activities. Occupational and

Table 4–1. Features of narcolepsy and idiopathic hypersomnia

	Narcolepsy	Idiopathic hypersomnia
Clinical feature		
Age at onset	Usually in adolescence	Usually in adolescence
Familial cases	Rare	Rare
EDS	Yes	Yes
Cataplexy	In 70%+ of cases	No
Sleep paralysis	Common	Less common
Hypnagogic hallucinations	Common	Less common
Total sleep time/24 hours	Normal	Increased
Nocturnal sleep fragmentation	Yes	No
Sleep-onset REM	Common	No
Test result		
Nocturnal polysomnogram	Sleep fragmentation	Increased sleep time
MSLT	Short latency, SOREMPs	Short latency; no SOREMPs
CSF hypocretin	Reduced or absent (in patients with cataplexy)	Normal

Note. EDS=excessive daytime sleepiness; REM=rapid eye movement; MSLT= multiple sleep latency test; SOREMPs=sleep-onset REM periods; CSF=cerebrospinal fluid.

social functioning may be severely affected by sleepiness. Nocturnal sleep time tends to be long, and patients are usually difficult to awaken in the morning, becoming irritable or even abusive in response to the efforts of others to rouse them. In some patients, this difficulty may be substantial and may include confusion, disorientation, and poor motor coordination, a condition sometimes termed "sleep drunkenness" (Roth et al. 1972). These patients often take naps, which may be prolonged but, in contrast to naps in narcolepsy, are usually nonrefreshing. No amount of sleep ameliorates the EDS. "Microsleeps," with or without automatic behavior, may occur throughout the day.

Polysomnographic studies of patients with idiopathic CNS hypersomnia usually reveal shortened initial sleep latency, increased total sleep time, and normal sleep architecture, in contrast to narcoleptic patients, who exhibit significant sleep fragmentation. Using quantitative electroencephalography, Sforza et al. (2000) found reduced sleep pressure, as evidenced by decreased slow-wave activity during the first two NREM episodes of nocturnal sleep, in patients with idiopathic hypersomnia. Mean sleep latency on MSLT is usually reduced, often in the 8–10-minute range but sometimes dramatically shorter. Also in contrast to narcolepsy, SOREMPs are not typically seen.

As with narcolepsy, other disorders producing EDS (such as insufficient sleep, sleep-related breathing disorders, PLMD, other sleep-fragmenting disorders, psychiatric diseases, and circadian rhythm disorders) must be ruled out before the diagnosis of idiopathic hypersomnia is made.

Recurrent Hypersomnias

Kleine-Levin syndrome. This uncommon disorder is a form of recurrent hypersomnia that occurs primarily in adolescents (Critchley 1967), with a male preponderance. It is characterized by the occurrence of episodes of EDS and is usually, but not invariably, accompanied by hyperphagia, aggressiveness, and hypersexuality. These episodes last for days to weeks and are separated by asymptomatic periods of weeks or months. During symptomatic periods, individuals sleep up to 18 hours per day and are usually drowsy (often to the degree of stupor), confused, and irritable the remainder of the time. During symptomatic episodes, polysomnographic studies show long total sleep time with high sleep efficiency and decreased slow-wave sleep. MSLT studies demonstrate short sleep latencies and SOREMPs (Rosenow et al. 2000).

The etiology of this syndrome remains obscure. Symptomatic cases of Kleine-Levin syndrome associated with structural brain lesions have been reported, but most cases are idiopathic. Single-photon emission computed tomography studies have demonstrated hypoperfusion in the thalamus in one patient and in the nondominant frontal lobe in another (Arias et al. 2002).

Menstrual-related hypersomnia. In this form of recurrent hypersomnia, EDS occurs during the several days prior to menstruation (Billiard et al. 1975; Sachs et al. 1982). The prevalence of this syndrome has not been well characterized. Likewise, the etiology is not known, but presumably the symptoms are related to hormonal changes. Some cases of menstrual-related hypersomnia have responded to the blocking of ovulation with estrogen and progesterone (birth control pills) (Bamford 1993).

Idiopathic recurring stupor. Numerous cases have been reported in which individuals (predominantly middle-aged males) are subject to stuporous episodes lasting from hours to days, in the absence of obvious toxic, metabolic, or structural cause. Episodes occur unpredictably, and the individuals are normal between episodes. Electroencephalographic data collected during symptomatic episodes have shown fast background activity in the 13–16 Hz range. Several of these patients have been shown to have elevated plasma and CSF levels of endozepine-4, an endogenous ligand with affinity for the benzodiazepine recognition site at the γ-aminobutyric acid type A receptor (Rothstein et al. 1992). Administration of flumazenil, a benzodiazepine antagonist, has produced transient awakening with normalization of the EEG profile (Lugaresi et al. 1998). In some cases, the episodes resolved spontaneously after several years. Similar cases have been reported in children (Soriani et al. 1997).

Nervous System Disorders and Excessive Daytime Sleepiness

EDS is often associated with disorders of the central or peripheral nervous system. It is a clinical feature of many toxic or metabolic encephalopathic processes. These disorders often present with other symptoms and signs, but EDS may dominate the picture, particularly in chronic cases. Structural brain lesions, including strokes, tumors, cysts, abscesses, hematomas, vascular malformations, hydrocephalus, and multiple sclerosis plaques, are known to produce EDS. Somnolence may result either from direct involvement of discrete brain regions (especially the brainstem reticular formation or midline diencephalic structures) or from effects on sleep continuity (for example, nocturnal seizure activity or sleep-related breathing disorders such as sleep apnea).

EDS is a frequent sequela of encephalitis or head trauma. Victims of "encephalitis lethargica," described by Von Economo in the early twentieth century, were found to have lesions in the midbrain, subthalamus, and hypothalamus. Additionally, posttraumatic narcolepsy with cataplexy is well documented (Francisco and Ivanhoe 1996). Epileptic patients may experience EDS as a consequence of medication effects or, less obviously, nocturnal seizure activity (Manni and Tartara 2000). EDS may be associated with numerous infectious agents affecting the CNS, including bacteria, viruses, fungi, and parasites. Perhaps the best known is trypanosomiasis, which is called "sleeping sickness" because of the prominent hypersomnia. Sleepiness may occur with acute infectious illness, even without direct invasion of the nervous system, and may be mediated by cytokines, including interferon, interleukins, and tumor necrosis factor (Toth and Opp 2002). EDS may also persist chronically after certain viral infections (Guilleminault and Mondini 1986).

Sleep disruption and EDS are also common in neurodegenerative disorders, including Parkinson's disease, Alzheimer's disease, and other dementias, as well as multiple system atrophy (Askenasy 1993; Chokroverty 1996; Trenkwalder 1998). Patients with neuromuscular disorders or peripheral neuropathies may also develop EDS due to associated central or obstructive sleep apnea, pain, or PLMD (George 2000). Patients with myotonic dystrophy often suffer from EDS, even in the absence of sleep-disordered breathing (Gibbs et al. 2002).

Finally, psychiatric illness, especially depression, is often accompanied by complaints of EDS. Indeed, tiredness, fatigue, or lack of energy are reported by an overwhelming majority of patients with major depression (Tylee et al. 1999). However, evaluation of true EDS with subjective rating scales and objective measures suggests that frank sleepiness or a high sleep propensity may be much less common than the complaint of fatigue or lack of energy. The few published studies evaluating objective measures of sleepiness (such as the MSLT) in depression suggest that only a minority of depressed patients have clinically important EDS and that the majority are in the normal range (Reynolds et al. 1982).

Management of Disorders of Excessive Daytime Sleepiness

Behavioral Treatment

In addition to the use of medications, the effective treatment of primary EDS conditions requires instituting structured and regular nocturnal sleep as well as structured daytime naps. A period of 8 hours or longer should be established for nocturnal sleep, with a consistent bedtime and time of morning awakening. Inadequate sleep duration, poor sleep environment, and fluctuating sleep-wake schedules can contribute substantially to daytime sleepiness, even in patients with primary sleep disorders. Moreover, shift work in any form is usually problematic. Additionally, in many EDS disorders, such as narcolepsy, scheduling two or more brief naps at regular times during the day is almost always necessary to further enhance daytime function. The importance of regular and adequate nocturnal and daytime sleep must always be emphasized with the patient.

Pharmacologic Treatment

Stimulants and Other Alerting Medications

Alerting agents provide a critical component of treatment for most patients with primary disorders of EDS (Mitler et al. 1994) (Table 4–2). Occasionally, patients may wish to avoid medications and instead may attempt to take extra naps during the day. This approach can be successful but usually fails to provide enough daytime alertness to function adequately. For most patients with narcolepsy, alerting agents do not yield a normal degree of daytime alertness but will nonetheless produce substantial improvement (Mitler et al. 1994). Clinically, the practice of combining two alerting agents of different chemical classes has been employed when a single agent is insufficient. This technique can be useful and is undergoing controlled evaluation in a large international trial with modafinil and sodium oxybate in narcolepsy.

Table 4–2. Common alerting agents for the treatment of excessive daytime sleepiness

Agent	Receptor	$T_{\frac{1}{2}}$ (h)	T_{max} (h)	Dose	Side effects
Modafinil	Unknown	15	2–4	100–400+ mg once daily or divided	Headache, nausea, anxiety, irritability
Amphetamines	Dopamine agonist	10 SR: 15+	2 SR: 8–10	5–60 mg divided	*Both amphetamines and methylphenidate:* headache, anxiety/irritability, increased BP, palpitation, appetite suppression, tremor, insomnia
Methylphenidate	Dopamine agonist	4 h SR: 8–10	2 SR: 5	5–60 mg divided	
Pemoline[a]	Dopamine agonist	12	2–4	18.75–112.5 mg daily or divided	As for amphetamines and methylphenidate, but milder
γ-Hydroxybutyrate	Inadequately characterized	2	1	6–9+ g liquid solution divided nightly	Sedation, nausea

Note. BP=blood pressure; SR=sustained release $T_{\frac{1}{2}}$=half-life; T_{max}=time to maximal concentration.
[a]Potentially hepatotoxic; frequent liver function monitoring required.

Modafinil. Modafinil is a wake-promoting therapeutic somewhat comparable to traditional stimulants in promoting alertness, but with a different mechanism of action. This mechanism is unknown, but modafinil appears to act more locally at hypothalamic regions and less globally on the CNS than the traditional stimulants (US Modafinil in Narcolepsy Multicenter Study Group 2000). The clinical duration of effect of modafinil may be longer because its serum half-life (12–15 hours) is longer than that of traditional stimulants. Modafinil has been evaluated extensively in the treatment of the EDS of narcolepsy, and in other sleep disorders manifesting EDS, and has been found to be useful in ameliorating EDS in these conditions (US Modafinil in Narcolepsy Multicenter Study Group 1998).

Sodium oxybate (GHB). Another agent that has been found to enhance alertness in narcolepsy is sodium oxybate, also known as γ-hydroxybutyrate (GHB). This agent has been explored extensively and found to be highly effective for the treatment of EDS in narcolepsy (Mamelak et al. 2004). The mechanism of action of the agent has been explored over many years, but how it effects improved alertness is unknown (Tunnicliff and Cash 2002). Data from multiple studies demonstrate that sodium oxybate imparts a degree of alertness similar to that of other agents and that its effect may be additive when used in combination with other stimulants (US Xyrem in Narcolepsy Multi-center Study Group 2002). Whether sodium oxybate will prove useful in other conditions of primary EDS is unknown.

Traditional stimulants. Commonly used traditional stimulants include methylphenidate, dextroamphetamine, and methamphetamine (Mitler et al. 1994). Other sympathomimetic amines and sustained-release preparations are available. Patients may experience negative effects with any alerting agent. Some patients report rebound hypersomnia (exacerbation of sleepiness) as the dose wears off. Tolerance (tachyphylaxis) to the alerting effect may occur with time in some patients. In cases of tolerance, switching to a different class of medication or providing a "drug holiday" can be useful.

Medications for Cataplexy (Anticataplectics)

Medications useful in the treatment of cataplexy usually also improve hypnagogic/hypnopompic hallucinations and sleep paralysis.

Sodium oxybate (GHB). In addition to its effect on EDS in narcolepsy, sodium oxybate is remarkably effective as an anticataplectic. It has been extensively evaluated as an anticataplectic agent over many years (US Xyrem in Narcolepsy Multi-center Study Group 2002). Additionally, GHB is effective in reducing nocturnal sleep disruptions and consolidating nocturnal sleep. Again, the mechanism of action of GHB in treating these symptoms is unknown (Tunnicliff and Cash 2002).

Antidepressants. Very low doses of tricyclic antidepressants (TCA) and typical antidepressant doses of selective serotonin reuptake inhibitors (SSRI), especially those with CNS noradrenergic activity, are also useful in treating cataplexy (Nishino and Mignot 1997). Tolerance to these traditional cataplexy medications can occur, requiring medication switch or drug holiday. Atomoxetine, venlafaxine, and other newer non-SSRI/non-tricyclic antidepressants have been reported in individual cases to provide effective treatment for cataplexy, although they have not yet been rigorously studied.

Pathophysiology of Narcolepsy

Narcolepsy Symptoms

The similarity between cataplexy and REM sleep atonia, the presence of frequent episodes of hypnagogic hallucinations and of sleep paralysis, and the propensity for narcolepsy patients to go directly from wakefulness into REM sleep suggest that narcolepsy is primarily a "disease of REM sleep" (Dement et al. 1966). This hypothesis may, however, be too simplistic, and it does not explain the presence of sleepiness during the day and the short latency to both NREM and REM sleep during nocturnal and nap recordings. A complementary hypothesis is that narcolepsy results from the disruption of the control mechanisms of both sleep and wakefulness or, in other words, from vigilance-state boundary problems (Broughton et al. 1986). According to this hypothesis, a cataplectic attack represents an intrusion of REM sleep atonia during wakefulness, and the hypnagogic hallucinations appear as dreamlike imagery taking place in the waking state, especially at sleep onset in patients who frequently have SOREMPs.

Cataplexy is associated with an inhibition of the monosynaptic H-reflex and the polysynaptic deep tendon reflexes (Guilleminault et al. 1974). In healthy subjects, it is only during REM sleep that the H-reflex is totally suppressed. This finding highlights the relationship between the inhibition of motor processes during REM sleep and the sudden atonia and areflexia seen during cataplexy. Studies in canine narcolepsy, however, suggest that the mechanisms for induction of cataplexy are different from those for REM sleep (Nishino et al. 2000a). Furthermore, an extended human study confirmed that cataplexy correlates much more highly with hypocretin deficiency (discussed below) than do other REM sleep–related phenomena (Mignot et al. 2002). Cataplexy may thus be viewed as a hypocretin-deficiency pathological phenomenon somewhat distinct from other REM-related symptoms. Patients with other sleep disorders such as sleep apnea, and even healthy individuals, can manifest SOREMPs, hypnagogic hallucinations, and sleep paralysis when their sleep-wake patterns are sufficiently disturbed. However, these subjects never develop cataplexy, further supporting the proposal that cataplexy is unrelated to other REM-associated symptoms (Aldrich et al. 1997; Bishop et al. 1996; Fukuda et al. 1987; Ohayon et al. 1996). Although cataplexy and REM sleep atonia have great similarity and possibly share a common executive system, the regulatory mechanisms of the two states are not necessarily identical. The mechanism of emotional triggering of cataplexy remains undetermined.

Narcolepsy, Human Leukocyte Antigen, and the Immune System

A remarkably high association of HLA with narcolepsy was discovered in the early 1980s (Juji et al. 1984). Since the time of this initial finding, a variety of research across multiple ethnic groups has corroborated the existence of this strong HLA association. The most specific marker of narcolepsy in a number of different ethnic groups studied to date is DQB1*0602 (Mignot 1998). This association is seen in an average of approximately 90% of those with unequivocal cataplexy (Mignot et al. 1997). Importantly, this association is substantially lower (only approximately 40%) in individuals who have received the diagnosis of narcolepsy but do not have cataplexy.

The strong association between HLA type and narcolepsy with cataplexy raises the possibility that narcolepsy is an autoimmune disease (Mignot et al. 1992). There is, however, no evidence of inflammatory processes or immune abnormalities associated with narcolepsy (Mignot et al. 1992). Studies have found no classical autoantibodies and no increase in oligoclonal CSF bands in individuals with narcolepsy (Fredrikson et al. 1990). Results of typical autoimmune pathology measures (erythrocyte sedimentation rates, serum immunoglobulin levels, C-reactive protein levels, complement levels, and lymphocyte subset ratios) are apparently normal in narcoleptic patients (Matsuki et al. 1988). In contrast, a variety of serological tests performed in narcoleptic patients and in age- and sex-matched control subjects yielded higher levels of antistreptolysin 0 and anti-DNase antibodies in patients than in control subjects (Billiard et al. 1989; Montplaisir et al. 1989). In view of these preliminary data, further exploration of possible immune-related dysfunction in narcolepsy is warranted.

Deficiency in Hypocretin (Orexin) Transmission in Canine and Human Narcolepsy

Narcolepsy Genes in Animal Models

Narcolepsy has been described in several animal species, including dogs, and most recently in genetically engineered mice models. Canine narcolepsy is a naturally occurring model, with both sporadic forms (17 breeds) and familial forms (Doberman, Labrador, and dachshund). In Doberman pinschers and Labrador retrievers, the disease is transmitted as a recessive autosomal trait with complete penetrance (Mignot et al. 1991).

In 1999, using positional cloning and gene targeting strategies, two groups independently revealed the pathogenesis of narcolepsy in animals. The lack of the hypothalamic neuropeptide hypocretin/orexin ligand (preprohypocretin/orexin gene knockout mice [Chemelli et al. 1999]) or mutations in one of the two hypocretin/orexin receptor genes (hypocretin receptor 2 [*hcrtr 2*] gene in autosomal recessive canine narcolepsy [Lin et al. 1999]) was observed to result in narcolepsy. Extensive screening in humans, especially in familial and early-onset narcolepsy, demonstrated that mutations in hypocretin-related genes are rare; only a single case with early onset (at age 6 months) was found to be associated with a single-point mutation in the preprohypocretin gene (Peyron et al. 2000).

Hypocretin Deficiency in Human Narcolepsy

Despite the lack of genetic abnormalities in the hypocretin system, the large majority (85%–90%) of patients with narcolepsy-cataplexy have low or undetectable hypocretin-1 ligand in their cerebrospinal fluid (Figure 4–1) (Nishino et al. 2000b, 2001b). This hypocretin deficiency is tightly associated with occurrence of cataplexy and HLA-DQ1*0602 positivity (Kanbayashi et al. 2002; Krahn et al. 2002; Mignot et al. 2002). Postmortem human studies, although using few brains, have confirmed hypocretin ligand deficiency (both hypocretin-1 and -2) in the narcoleptic brain (Figure 4–1) (Peyron et al. 2000; Thannickal et al. 2000). Hypocretin deficiency has also been observed in sporadic cases of canine narcolepsy (7 of 7 animals studied; the results of 4 cases are reported), suggesting that the pathophysiology in these animals mirrors that of most human cases (Ripley et al. 2001a).

The establishment of CSF hypocretin measurement as a new diagnostic tool in human narcolepsy is encouraging. Although positive predictive value is not 100%, low CSF hypocretin-1 levels are very specific for narcolepsy when compared with other sleep or neurologic disorders (Figure 4–2) (Kanbayashi et al. 2002; Mignot et al. 2002; Ripley et al. 2001b). Previously, no specific and sensitive diagnostic test for narcolepsy based on the pathophysiology of the disease was available, and the final diagnosis was often delayed for several years after the onset (typically during adolescence) of the disease (Alaila 1992). Many

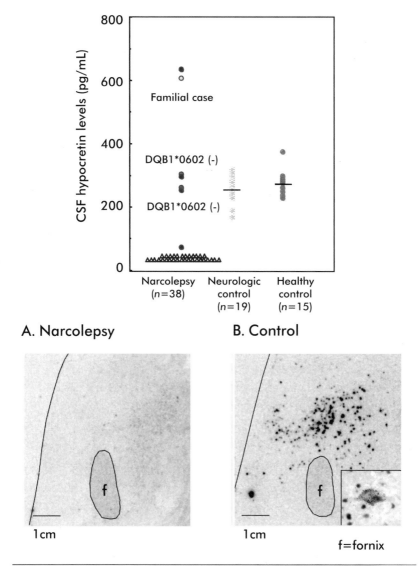

Figure 4–1. CSF hypocretin levels in narcoleptic and control subjects (top panel). Hypocretin mRNA in situ hybridization in the hypothalamus of narcoleptic and control subjects (bottom panels).

Top: CSF hypocretin-1 levels are undetectably low in most narcoleptic subjects (84.2%). Note that two HLA DQB1*0602 negative cases and one familial case have normal or high CSF hypocretin-1 levels. Data from Nishino et al. 2001b. **Bottom:** Preprohypocretin transcripts are detected in the hypothalamus of control (**B**) but not narcoleptic (**A**) subjects. Melanin-concentrating hormone transcripts are detected in the same region in both control and narcoleptic sections (data not shown). *Source.* Modified from Peyron et al. 2000.

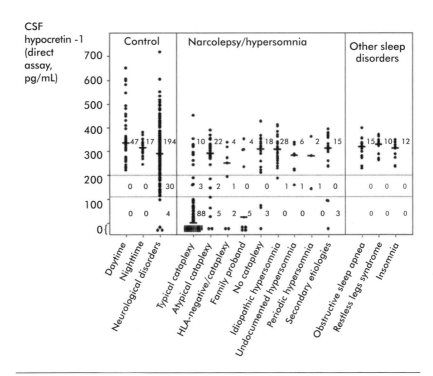

Figure 4–2. CSF hypocretin-1 levels across various disease categories. Each dot represents a single patient. Hypocretin-1 levels were determined with a direct assay without prior extraction. Hypocretin-1 values below 110 pg/mL were determined to be diagnostic for narcolepsy. Concentrations above 200 pg/mL best determine healthy control values. The number of patients with hypocretin values below or equal to 110 pg/mL, above 200 pg/mL and between these two values is indicated for each category. CSF = cerebrospinal fluid; HLA = human leukocyte antigen.
Source. Modified from Mignot et al. 2002.

patients with narcolepsy and related EDS disorders are therefore likely to obtain immediate benefit from this new specific diagnostic test. In addition, hypocretin agonists may be promising in the treatment of narcolepsy.

Hypocretin/orexin and Sleep Physiology

Hypocretins/orexins were identified by two independent research groups in 1998, one year prior to the cloning of the canine narcolepsy gene. One group called the peptides *hypocretin* because of their primary hypothalamic localization and similarities with the hormone secretin (De Lecea et al. 1998). The other group called the molecules *orexin* after observing that central administration of these peptides increased appetite in rats (Sakurai et al. 1998). Hypocretin-1 and -2 are produced exclusively by a well-defined group of neurons localized in the lateral hypothalamus. The neurons project to the olfactory bulb, cerebral cortex, thalamus, hypothalamus, and brainstem, particularly the locus coeruleus (LC), raphe nucleus, and cholinergic nuclei and cholinoceptive sites (such as pontine reticular formation), thought to be important for sleep regulation (Peyron et al. 1998).

The hypocretin system is a major excitatory system that affects the activity of monoaminergic (dopamine, norepinephrine, serotonin, and histamine) and cholinergic systems with major effects on vigilance states (Taheri et al. 2002; Willie et al. 2001). It is therefore likely that a deficiency in hypocretin neurotransmission induces an imbalance between these classical neurotransmitter systems, with primary effects on sleep-state organization and vigilance. Indeed, dopamine and/or norepinephrine contents have been reported to be high in several brain structures in narcoleptic Dobermans and in human narcolepsy postmortem brains (Nishino and Mignot 1997). These changes in humans are possibly due to compensatory mechanisms, because drugs that enhance dopaminergic neurotransmission (such as amphetamine-like stimulants and modafinil for EDS) and norepinephrine neurotransmission (such as noradrenaline uptake blockers for cataplexy) are commonly used (Nishino and Mignot 1997).

Histamine is another monoamine implicated in the control of vigilance, and the histaminergic system is also likely to indirectly mediate the wake-promoting effects of hypocretin (Eriksson et al. 2001; Huang et al. 2001; Yamanaka et al. 2002). Interestingly, brain histamine contents both in *hcrtr*-2 gene–mutated and in ligand-deficient narcoleptic dogs are dramatically reduced (Nishino et al. 2001a). The involvement of the histaminergic system in the pathophysiology of narcolepsy and therapeutic applications of histaminergic compounds (Tedford et al. 1999) should be further studied.

Studies of animal hypocretin system function suggest that basic hypocretin neurotransmission fluctuates across the 24-hour period and slowly builds up during the active period (Fujiki et al.

2001; Yoshida et al. 2001; Zeitzer et al. 2003). Adrenergic LC neurons are typical wake-active neurons involved in vigilance control, and it has been recently demonstrated that basic firing activity of wake-active LC neurons also significantly fluctuates across various circadian times (Aston-Jones et al. 2001). Several acute manipulations, such as exercise, low glucose utilization in the brain, and forced wakefulness, increase hypocretin levels (Willie et al. 2001; Wu et al. 2002; Yoshida et al. 2001). It is therefore hypothesized that a buildup or acute increase of hypocretin levels may counteract the homeostatic sleep propensity that typically increases during the daytime and during forced wakefulness (Yoshida et al. 2001; Zeitzer et al. 2003). Because of the lack of increase in hypocretin tone, narcoleptic subjects may not be able to stay awake for a prolonged period and do not respond to various alerting stimuli. Conversely, the reduction of the hypocretin tone at sleep onset may contribute to the profound deep sleep that normally inhibits REM sleep at sleep onset, and the lack of this system in narcolepsy may allow the occurrence of REM sleep at sleep onset.

Summary

Excessive daytime sleepiness is a prevalent problem in medical practice and in society in general. It exacts a great cost in terms of quality of life, personal and public safety, and productivity. The causes of EDS are myriad, and a careful evaluation is needed to determine the cause in an individual case. Although much progress has been made in discovering the pathophysiology of narcolepsy, much more remains to be understood, and far less is known about other primary conditions of EDS. Several methods have been developed to assess EDS, although each of them has limitations. Treatment is available for the great majority of individuals with excessive daytime sleepiness.

References

Alaila SL: Life effects of narcolepsy: measures of negative impact, social support and psychological well-being, in Psychosocial Aspects of Narcolepsy (Loss, Grief and Care Series, No. 3). Edited by Goswanmi M, Pollak CP, Cohen FL, et al. New York, Haworth, 1992, pp 1–22

Aldrich MS: The clinical spectrum of narcolepsy and idiopathic hypersomnia. Neurology 46:393–401, 1996

Aldrich MS, Chervin RD, Malow BA: Value of the Multiple Sleep Latency Test (MSLT) for the diagnosis of narcolepsy. Sleep 20:620–629, 1997

American Psychiatric Association: Diagnostic and Statistical Manual of Mental Disorders, 4th Edition, Text Revision. Washington, DC, American Psychiatric Publishing, 2000

American Sleep Disorders Association: International Classification of Sleep Disorders, Revised: Diagnostic and Coding Manual. Rochester, MN, American Sleep Disorders Association, 1997

Arias M, Crespo Iglesias JM, Perez J, et al: [Kleine-Levin syndrome: contribution of brain SPECT in diagnosis] (Spanish). Rev Neurol 35:531–533, 2002

Askenasy JJ: Sleep in Parkinson's disease. Acta Neurol Scand 87:167–170, 1993

Aston-Jones G, Chen S, Zhu Y, et al: A neural circuit for circadian regulation of arousal. Nature Neurosci 4:732–738, 2001

Bamford CR: Menstrual-associated sleep disorder: an unusual hypersomniac variant associated with both menstruation and amenorrhea with a possible link to prolactin and metoclopramide. Sleep 16:484–486, 1993

Bassetti C, Aldrich MS: Idiopathic hypersomnia: a series of 42 patients. Brain 120:1423–1435, 1997

Beusterien KM, Rogers AE, Walsleben JA, et al: Health-related quality of life effects of modafinil for treatment of narcolepsy. Sleep 22:757–765, 1999

Billiard M, Dauvilliers Y: Idiopathic hypersomnia. Sleep Med Rev 5:349–358, 2001

Billiard M, Guilleminault C, Dement WC: A menstruation-linked periodic hypersomnia: Kleine-Levin syndrome or a new clinical entity? Neurology 25:436–443, 1975

Billiard M, Laaberki MF, Reygrobellet C, et al: Elevated antibodies to streptococcal antigens in narcoleptic subjects (abstract). Sleep Res 18:201, 1989

Bishop C, Rosenthal L, Helmus T, et al: The frequency of multiple sleep onset REM periods among subjects with no excessive daytime sleepiness. Sleep 19:727–730, 1996

Broughton R, Valley V, Aguirre M, et al: Excessive daytime sleepiness and pathophysiology of narcolepsy-cataplexy: a laboratory perspective. Sleep 9:105–215, 1986

Bruck D, Parkes JD: A comparison of idiopathic hypersomnia and narcolepsy-cataplexy using self report measures and sleep diary data. J Neurol Neurosurg Psychiatr 60:576–578, 1996

Chemelli RM, Willie JT, Sinton CM, et al: Narcolepsy in orexin knockout mice: molecular genetics of sleep regulation. Cell 98:437–451, 1999

Chokroverty S: Sleep and degenerative neurologic disorders. Neurol Clin 14:807–826, 1996

Critchley M: [The syndrome of hypersomnia and periodical megaphagia in the adult male (Kleine-Levin): what is its natural course?] (French). Rev Neurol (Paris) 116:647–650, 1967

De Lecea L, Kilduff TS, Peyron C, et al: The hypocretins: hypothalamus-specific peptides with neuroexcitatory activity. Proc Natl Acad Sci USA 95:322–327, 1998

Dement W, Rechtschaffen A, Gulevich G: The nature of the narcoleptic sleep attack. Neurology 16:18–33, 1966

Eriksson KS, Sergeeva O, Brown RE, et al: Orexin/hypocretin excites the histaminergic neurons of the tuberomammillary nucleus. J Neurosci 21:9273–9279, 2001

Faull KF, Guilleminault C, Berger PA, et al: Cerebrospinal fluid monoamine metabolites in narcolepsy and hypersomnia. Ann Neurol 13:258–263, 1983

Faull KF, Thiemann S, King RJ, et al: Monoamine interactions in narcolepsy and hypersomnia: a preliminary report. Sleep 9:246–249, 1986

Francisco GE, Ivanhoe CB: Successful treatment of post-traumatic narcolepsy with methylphenidate: a case report. Am J Phys Med Rehabil 75:63–65, 1996

Fredrikson S, Carlander B, Billiard M, et al: CSF immune variables in patients with narcolepsy. Acta Neurol Scand 81:253–254, 1990

Fujiki N, Yoshida Y, Ripley B, et al: Changes in CSF hypocretin-1 (orexin A) levels in rats across 24 hours and in response to food deprivation. Neuroreport 12:993–997, 2001

Fukuda K, Miyasita A, Inugami M, et al: High prevalence of isolated sleep paralysis: Kanashibari phenomenon in Japan. Sleep 10:279–286, 1987

Gelb M, Guilleminault C, Kraemer H, et al: Stability of cataplexy over several months: information for the design of therapeutic trials. Sleep 17:265–273, 1994

George CFP: Neuromuscular disorders, in Principles and Practice of Sleep Medicine, 3rd Edition. Edited by Kryger MH, Roth T, Dement WC. Philadelphia, PA, WB Saunders, 2000, pp 1087–1092

Gibbs JW 3rd, Ciafaloni E, Radtke RA: Excessive daytime somnolence and increased rapid eye movement pressure in myotonic dystrophy. Sleep 25:672–675, 2002

Guilleminault C, Mondini S: Mononucleosis and chronic daytime sleepiness: a long-term follow-up study. Arch Intern Med 146:1333–1335, 1986

Guilleminault C, Wilson RA, Dement WC: A study on cataplexy. Arch Neurol 31:255–261, 1974

Guilleminault C, Stoohs R, Clerk A, et al: A cause of excessive daytime sleepiness: the upper airway resistance syndrome. Chest 104:781–787, 1993

Honda Y: Clinical features of narcolepsy: Japanese experiences, in HLA in Narcolepsy. Edited by Honda Y, Juji T. Berlin, Springer-Verlag, 1988, pp 24–57

Huang ZL, Qu WM, Li WD, et al: Arousal effect of orexin A depends on activation of the histaminergic system. Proc Natl Acad Sci USA 98:9965–9970, 2001

Johns MW: A new method for measuring daytime sleepiness: the Epworth Sleepiness Scale. Sleep 14:540–545, 1991

Juji T, Satake M, Honda Y, et al: HLA antigens in Japanese patients with narcolepsy: all the patients were DR2 positive. Tissue Antigens 24:316–319, 1984

Kanbayashi T, Inoue Y, Chiba S, et al: CSF hypocretin-1 (orexin-A) concentrations in narcolepsy with and without cataplexy and idiopathic hypersomnia. J Sleep Res 11:91–93, 2002

Krahn LE, Pankratz VS, Oliver L, et al: Hypocretin (orexin) levels in cerebrospinal fluid of patients with narcolepsy: relationship to cataplexy and HLA DQB1*0602 status. Sleep 25:733–736, 2002

Lin L, Faraco J, Li R, et al: The sleep disorder canine narcolepsy is caused by a mutation in the hypocretin (orexin) receptor 2 gene. Cell 98:365–376, 1999

Lugaresi E, Montagna P, Tinuper P, et al: Endozepine stupor: recurring stupor linked to endozepine-4 accumulation. Brain 121:127–133, 1998

Mamelak M, Black J, Montplaisir J, et al: A pilot study on the effects of sodium oxybate on sleep architecture and daytime alertness in narcolepsy. Sleep 27:1327–1334, 2004

Manni R, Tartara A: Evaluation of sleepiness in epilepsy. Clin Neurophysiol 111 (suppl 2): S111–S114, 2000

Matsuki K, Juji T, Honda Y: Immunological features of narcolepsy in Japan, in HLA in Narcolepsy. Edited by Honda Y, Juji T. Berlin, Springer-Verlag, 1988, pp 150–157

Mignot E: Genetic and familial aspects of narcolepsy. Neurology 50 (suppl 1):S16–S22, 1998

Mignot E, Wang C, Rattazzi C, et al: Genetic linkage of autosomal recessive canine narcolepsy with a mu immunoglobulin heavy-chain switch-like segment. Proc Natl Acad Sci USA 88:3475–3478, 1991

Mignot E, Guilleminault C, Grumet FC, et al: Is narcolepsy an autoimmune disease? In Proceedings of the Third Milano International Symposium, September 18–19, "Sleep, Hormones, and the Immune System." Edited by Smirne S, Francesci M, Ferini-Strambi L, Zucconi M. Milan, Masson, 1992, pp 29–38

Mignot E, Hayduk R, Black J, et al: HLA Class II studies in 509 narcoleptic patients. Sleep Res 26:433, 1997

Mignot E, Lammers GJ, Ripley B, et al: The role of cerebrospinal fluid hypocretin measurement in the diagnosis of narcolepsy and other hypersomnias. Arch Neurol 59:1553–1562, 2002

Mitler MM, Aldrich MS, Koob GF, et al: Narcolepsy and its treatment with stimulants: ASDA standards of practice. Sleep 17:352–371, 1994

Montplaisir J, Poirier G: HLA in disorders of excessive sleepiness without cataplexy in Canada, in HLA in Narcolepsy. Edited by Honda Y, Juji T. Berlin, Springer-Verlag, 1988, pp 186–190

Montplaisir J, De Champlain J, Young SN, et al: Narcolepsy and idiopathic hypersomnia: biogenic amines and related compounds in CSF. Neurology 32:1299–1302, 1982

Montplaisir J, Poirier G, Lapierre O, et al: Streptococcal antibodies in narcolepsy and idiopathic hypersomnia. Sleep Res 18:271, 1989

National Sleep Foundation: Sleep in America Poll 2002. Available at: http://www.sleepfoundation.org/2002poll.cfm. Accessed March 2005.

National Sleep Foundation: Sleep in America Poll 2003. Available at: http://www.sleepfoundation.org/2003poll.cfm. Accessed March 2005.

Nishino S, Mignot E: Pharmacological aspects of human and canine narcolepsy. Prog Neurobiol 52:27–78, 1997

Nishino S, Riehl J, Hong J, et al: Is narcolepsy REM sleep disorder? Analysis of sleep abnormalities in narcoleptic Dobermans. Neurosci Res 38:437–446, 2000a

Nishino S, Ripley B, Overeem S, et al: Hypocretin (orexin) deficiency in human narcolepsy. Lancet 355:39–40, 2000b

Nishino S, Fujiki N, Ripley B, et al: Decreased brain histamine contents in hypocretin/orexin receptor-2 mutated narcoleptic dogs. Neurosci Lett 313:125–128, 2001a

Nishino S, Ripley B, Overeem S, et al: Low CSF hypocretin (orexin) and altered energy homeostasis in human narcolepsy. Ann Neurol 50:381–388, 2001b

Ohayon MM, Priest RG, Caulet M, et al: Hypnagogic and hypnopompic hallucinations: pathological phenomena? Br J Psychiatry 169:459–467, 1996

Ohayon MM, Priest RG, Zulley J, et al: Prevalence of narcolepsy symptomatology and diagnosis in the European general population. Neurology 58:1826–1833, 2002

Overeem S, Mignot E, van Dijk JG, et al: Narcolepsy: clinical features, new pathophysiological insights, and future perspectives. J Clin Neurophysiol 18:78–105, 2001

Peyron C, Tighe DK, van den Pol AN, et al: Neurons containing hypocretin (orexin) project to multiple neuronal systems. J Neurosci 18:9996–10015, 1998

Peyron C, Faraco J, Rogers W, et al: A mutation in a case of early onset narcolepsy and a generalized absence of hypocretin peptides in human narcoleptic brains. Nat Med 6:991–997, 2000

Reynolds CF 3rd, Coble PA, Kupfer DJ, et al: Application of the Multiple Sleep Latency Test in disorders of excessive sleepiness. Electroencephalogr Clin Neurophysiol 53:443–452, 1982

Ripley B, Fujiki N, Okura M, et al: Hypocretin levels in sporadic and familial cases of canine narcolepsy. Neurobiol Dis 8:525–534, 2001a

Ripley B, Overeem S, Fujiki N, et al: CSF hypocretin levels in various neurological conditions: low levels in narcolepsy and Guillain-Barre syndrome (abstract). Sleep 24:A322, 2001b

Rosenow F, Kotagal P, Cohen BH, et al: Multiple Sleep Latency Test and polysomnography in diagnosing Kleine-Levin syndrome and periodic hypersomnia. J Clin Neurophysiol 17:519–522, 2000

Roth B: Narcolepsy and hypersomnia: review and classification of 642 personally observed cases. Schweiz Arch Neurol Neurochir Psychiatr 119:31–41, 1976

Roth B, Nevsimalova S, Rechtschaffen A: Hypersomnia with "sleep drunkenness." Arch Gen Psychiatry 26:456–462, 1972

Rothstein JD, Guidotti A, Tinuper P, et al: Endogenous benzodiazepine receptor ligands in idiopathic recurring stupor. Lancet 340:1002–1004, 1992

Sachs C, Persson H, Hagenfeldt K: Menstruation-associated periodic hypersomnia: a case study with successful treatment. Neurology 32:1376–1379, 1982

Sakurai T, Amemiya A, Ishii M, et al: Orexins and orexin receptors: a family of hypothalamic neuropeptides and G protein-coupled receptors that regulate feeding behavior. Cell 92:573–585, 1998

Sforza E, Gaudreau H, Petit D, et al: Homeostatic sleep regulation in patients with idiopathic hypersomnia. Clin Neurophysiol 111:277–282, 2000

Soriani S, Carrozzi M, De Carlo L, et al: Endozepine stupor in children. Cephalalgia 17:658–661, 1997

Taheri S, Zeitzer JM, Mignot E: The role of hypocretins (orexins) in sleep regulation and narcolepsy. Annu Rev Neurosci 25:283–313, 2002

Tedford CE, Edgar DM, Seidel WF, et al: Effects of a novel, selective, and potent histamine H_3 receptor antagonist, GT-2332, on rat sleep/wakefulness and canine cataplexy (abstract). Abstr Soc Neurosci 25:1134, 1999

Thannickal TC, Moore RY, Nienhuis R, et al: Reduced number of hypocretin neurons in human narcolepsy. Neuron 27:469–474, 2000

Toth LA, Opp MR: Sleep and infection, in Sleep Medicine. Edited by Lee-Chiong TL, Sateia MJ, Carskadon MA. Philadelphia, PA, Hanley and Belfus, 2002, pp 77–83

Trenkwalder C: Sleep dysfunction in Parkinson's disease. Clin Neurosci 5:107–114, 1998

Tunnicliff G, Cash CD: Gamma-hydroxybutyrate: Molecular, Functional and Clinical Aspects. New York, Taylor and Francis, 2002

Tylee A, Gastpar M, Lepine JP, et al: DEPRES II (Depression Research in European Society II): a patient survey of the symptoms, disability and current management of depression in the community. DEPRES Steering Committee. Int Clin Psychopharmacol 14:139–151, 1999

US Modafinil in Narcolepsy Multicenter Study Group: Randomized trial of modafinil for the treatment of pathological somnolence in narcolepsy. Ann Neurol 43:88–97, 1998

US Modafinil in Narcolepsy Multicenter Study Group: Randomized trial of modafinil as a treatment for the excessive daytime somnolence of narcolepsy. Neurology 54:1166–1175, 2000

US Xyrem in Narcolepsy Multi-center Study Group: A randomized, double blind, placebo-controlled multicenter trial comparing the effects of three doses of orally administered sodium oxybate with placebo for the treatment of narcolepsy. Sleep 25:42–49, 2002

Willie JT, Chemelli RM, Sinton CM, et al: To eat or to sleep? Orexin in the regulation of feeding and wakefulness. Annu Rev Neurosci 24:429–458, 2001

Wu MF, John J, Maidment N, et al: Hypocretin release in normal and narcoleptic dogs after food and sleep deprivation, eating, and movement. Am J Physiol Regul Integr Comp Physiol 283:R1079–R1086, 2002

Yamanaka A, Tsujino N, Funahashi H, et al: Orexins activate histaminergic neurons via the orexin 2 receptor. Biochem Biophys Res Commun 290:1237–1245, 2002

Yoshida Y, Fujiki N, Nakajima T, et al: Fluctuation of extracellular hypo-cretin-1 (orexin A) levels in the rat in relation to the light-dark cycle and sleep-wake activities. Eur J Neurosci 14:1075–1081, 2001

Zeitzer JM, Buckmaster CL, Parker KJ, et al: Circadian and homeostatic regulation of hypocretin in a primate model: implications for the consolidation of wakefulness. J Neurosci 23:3555–3560, 2003

Chapter 5

Restless Legs Syndrome

John W. Winkelman, M.D., Ph.D.

Restless legs syndrome (RLS) is a sensorimotor disorder that is generally not appropriately diagnosed or treated by the medical community because of nonchalance toward insomnia, inadequate awareness of RLS symptoms, and ignorance of optimal therapeutic approaches. Ignorance regarding RLS is surprising given that it was first recognized and described over 300 years ago.

For psychiatrists, RLS is an important topic because it is one of the most common treatable causes of insomnia (particularly in elderly persons), it is in the differential diagnosis of a number of psychiatric illnesses and iatrogenic states, and it is treated with medications that are commonly used in psychiatric practice. Furthermore, clinicians in other specialties within medicine may refer patients with RLS for evaluation, believing the symptoms of RLS to be psychiatric in nature.

Sir Thomas Willis first described the symptoms of RLS in 1672, reporting, "[W]herefore to some, when being a Bed they betake themselves to sleep, presently in the Arms and Leggs Leapings and Contractions of the Tendons, and so great a Restlessness and Tossing of their Members ensure, that the diseased are no more able to sleep, than if they were in a Place of the greatest Torture" (Winkelmann 1999). Little further description appeared until 1944, when Karl Ekbom made his classic observations of this disorder. At that time, the cardinal symptoms of the disorder became well established, the familial pattern was first described, and the possible role of iron in the pathogenesis of RLS was identified. Treatment has evolved dramatically in subsequent years.

Essential diagnostic criteria for RLS were first established in 1995 by consensus of the International Restless Legs Syndrome

Study Group (Walters 1995). These were recently modified at a National Institutes of Health consensus conference, although the general intent and form of the original criteria were maintained (Allen et al. 2003). These criteria (Table 5–1) are now used in both clinical trials and genetic research with RLS patients. No diagnostic criteria for RLS exist in DSM-IV-TR (American Psychiatric Association 2000), where it is characterized as *dyssomnia not otherwise specified.*

Diagnosis

According to the modified consensus criteria (Allen et al. 2003; see Table 5–1), the first essential criterion for a diagnosis of RLS is "an urge to move the legs, usually accompanied or caused by uncomfortable and unpleasant sensations in the legs." The disorder gets its name from this symptom, and it is the central aspect of the disorder. However, the limitations of the language of sensory experiences can make the diagnosis more difficult, as the restlessness and accompanying dysesthesia of RLS are described by patients in a variety of ways. Individuals classically describe the feeling as "achy" or "creepy-crawly," and although they often use descriptions that locate the sensations as deep in the leg ("electric," "a coiled spring," "something running down my veins,") they may also use words that refer to superficial sensations (e.g., "itchy"). Many individuals will report that the feeling is frankly painful, which may initiate an evaluation (and sometimes even surgical treatment) for a vascular or an orthopedic-based pain disorder. Not all patients will report both aspects of RLS (restlessness and dysesthesia) with equal emphasis, and some will report only one or the other aspect. Psychiatrists are familiar with restlessness in the context of akathisia, from which this aspect of RLS can be difficult to distinguish.

The dependence of the restlessness and dysesthesia on immobility is required by the second diagnostic criterion: "the urge to move or unpleasant sensations begin or worsen during periods of rest or inactivity such as lying or sitting." The majority of the clinical consequences of RLS are due to this aspect of the disorder, in that the predominant presenting complaint in those with RLS is of sleep disturbance, which is certainly a period of rest while lying down. RLS patients not only report symptoms while attempting to sleep, but may also report interference with reading, watching TV, and

Table 5–1.   Essential diagnostic criteria for restless legs syndrome

1. An urge to move the legs, usually accompanied or caused by uncomfortable and unpleasant sensations in the legs, is present. (Sometimes the urge to move is present without the uncomfortable sensations, and sometimes the arms or other body parts are involved in addition to the legs.)
2. The urge to move or unpleasant sensations begin or worsen during periods of rest or inactivity such as lying or sitting.
3. The urge to move or unpleasant sensations are partially or totally relieved by movement, such as walking or stretching, at least as long as the activity continues.
4. The urge to move or unpleasant sensations are worse in the evening or night than during the day or only occur in the evening or night. (When symptoms are very severe, the worsening at night may not be noticeable but must have been previously present.)

Source.   Reprinted from Allen RP et al: "Restless Legs Syndrome: Diagnostic Criteria, Special Considerations, and Epidemiology." *Sleep Medicine* 4:101–119, 2003. ©2003. Used with permission from Elsevier.

long car or plane travel. This time- and position-dependent aspect of RLS has allowed the symptom to be studied in a scientific and objective fashion, to some degree counteracting the ambiguous and subjective nature of the complaint. Montplaisir and colleagues (Michaud et al. 2002a) developed the Suggested Immobilization Test (SIT), in which the individual assumes a lying position with outstretched legs for 1 hour and is told not to move the legs unless necessary. Every 5 minutes, the individual rates his or her sensory discomfort, and measures of leg restlessness are made by surface electromyographic recordings from the anterior tibialis muscle. As can be seen from Figure 5–1, leg discomfort is significantly greater in RLS patients than in non-RLS control subjects within 10 minutes on the SIT, and leg discomfort continues to differentiate the two groups over time. This sensory discomfort differentiates RLS patients from control subjects with greater than 80% accuracy in SIT data (Michaud et al. 2002b), although this is not a substantial surprise given that an RLS diagnosis depends on this complaint.

The third criterion, that "the urge to move or unpleasant sensations are partially or totally relieved by movement, such as walking or stretching, at least as long as the activity continues," is

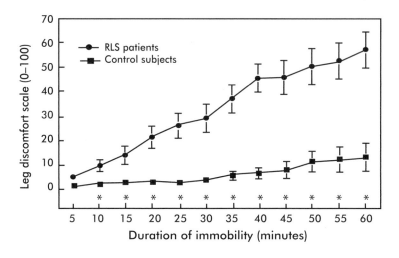

Figure 5–1. Relationship between SIT duration and mean (±SEM) leg discomfort scores in RLS patients and healthy control subjects.
RLS=restless legs syndrome; SIT=Suggested Immobilization Test.
*Significant contrasts at $P<0.05$.
Source. From Michaud M et al: "Effects of Immobility on Sensory and Motor Symptoms of Restless Legs Syndrome." *Movement Disorders* 17:112–115. ©2002. Reprinted with permission of Wiley-Liss, a subsidiary of John Wiley & Sons, Inc.

a corollary of the second criterion, and it can be extremely helpful in distinguishing RLS from other disorders characterized by dysesthesia or pain. RLS patients may move excessively in bed while awake (disturbing the bedpartner) or may need to interrupt activities requiring immobility to relieve the sensations. Such movement has both voluntary and involuntary aspects; movement is described as irrepressible, but it can be delayed or potentially avoided by distraction. While the patient is asleep, as described below, or is attempting to avoid movement (as in the SIT), characteristic movements of the legs appear (periodic leg movements of sleep or while awake) with a distinctive pattern and distribution. For some individuals, superficial stimulation of the legs by rubbing them or taking hot baths may bring relief, consistent with a "gating" of the RLS discomfort by these countermeasures. Other disorders that produce pain in the extremities (e.g., neuropathic pain, arthritis) are not as thoroughly (or not at all) relieved by movement, and thus can be excluded on this basis.

The fourth criterion is one of the most interesting, pathognomonic, and troublesome aspects of RLS: "the urge to move or unpleasant sensations are worse in the evening or night than during the day or only occur in the evening or night." For most patients, RLS is usually most severe between 8:00 P.M. and 4:00 A.M. and is least bothersome between 8:00 A.M. and noon. Worsening of RLS at night could potentially be due to the absence of distraction, the lying position, or accumulated wakefulness. However, studies using the constant routine protocol, in which individuals are kept awake for 30–40 hours, have demonstrated conclusively that RLS symptoms worsen at night, associated with a fall in body temperature and a rise in melatonin levels, and improve the following day (after sleep deprivation) even when the patient is kept in a reclining position, in an environment free of time cues, and under constant levels of stimulation (Michaud et al. 2004).

Consequences

The most disturbing consequences of RLS are difficulties with sleep onset and maintenance. Sleep disturbance in RLS is a result of the combination of its essential elements: appearance of RLS with immobility, its improvement with movement, and the nocturnal exacerbation of dysesthesia and restlessness. Individuals with RLS have among the worst sleep observed among the primary sleep disorders. Total sleep times of 4 hours are not uncommon in clinical samples of patients with moderate to severe RLS. Because of the daily appearance of symptoms within limited hours, some patients may attempt to sleep outside of the times during which their RLS is most severe. A report of optimal sleep after 4:00 A.M. in an elderly individual (in which the optimal sleep is usually advanced to the early evening hours) is strongly suggestive of RLS. However, excessive daytime sleepiness is usually not a substantial complaint in those with RLS, and the ability to nap during the day is often impaired because of restlessness in those with severe RLS.

Once asleep, roughly 80% of RLS patients will have periodic limb movements of sleep (PLMS), which are repetitive, brief (0.5–5.0 seconds) stereotyped movements of the foot and leg, appearing at roughly 20-second intervals (Michaud et al. 2002b) (Figure 5–2).

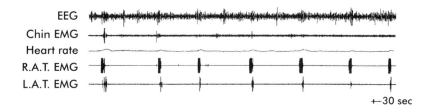

Figure 5–2. Polysomnographic recording of periodic limb movements of sleep.

EEG=electroencephalogram; EMG=electromyogram; R.A.T.=right anterior tibialis; L.A.T.=left anterior tibialis.

Source. Reprinted with permission of The McGraw-Hill Co. from Czeisler CA et al: "Sleep Disorders," in *Harrison's Principles of Internal Medicine,* 16th Ed. Edited by Kasper DL et al. New York, McGraw-Hill Professional, 2004, pp 153–162.

Such movements may be subtle or gross, can be associated with arousal from sleep, and produce movement-associated elevations in heart rate and blood pressure (Winkelman 1999). More than 5 such movements per hour of sleep is considered abnormal, and RLS patients often have more than 40 per hour. However, given the high prevalence of PLMS in the general population (and elevated rates in a number of specific disorders), polysomnography to document PLMS is not a specific enough diagnostic tool to be warranted in RLS patients (Montplaisir et al. 2000). Such involuntary leg movements can also occur during waking in RLS (periodic limb movements of wake), particularly during periods of immobility (or during the SIT) (Michaud et al. 2002a) (Figure 5–3).

RLS is associated with a substantial risk of elevated depression scores or reports of depressed mood (depending on the measurement used) in both epidemiologic and case-control studies, even when controlled for confounding disorders (Ulfberg et al. 2001). In the best study, which used face-to-face interviews to make an RLS diagnosis and the Center for Epidemiologic Studies Depression Scale (CES-D) to measure mood, men with RLS had 13 times the risk of elevated depression scores compared with men without RLS (Rothdach et al. 2000). Risk for depression in women was not observed in that study. Similarly, studies of quality of life measures demonstrate multiple impairments (Hening et al. 2004).

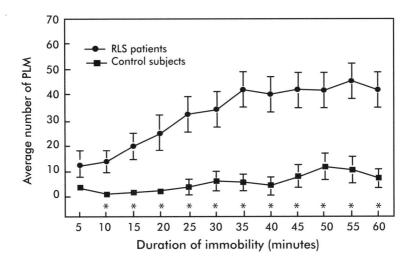

Figure 5–3. Relationship between SIT duration and average number (±SEM) of PLM per 5 minutes in RLS patients and healthy control subjects. PLM=periodic limb movements; RLS=restless legs syndrome; SIT=Suggested Immobilization Test.
*Significant contrasts at $P<0.05$.
Source. From Michaud M et al: "Effects of Immobility on Sensory and Motor Symptoms of Restless Legs Syndrome." *Movement Disorders* 17:112–115. ©2002. Reprinted with permission of Wiley-Liss, a subsidiary of John Wiley & Sons, Inc.

Prevalence and Clinical Course

A number of questionnaire-based estimates of RLS have been performed (Ohayon and Roth 2002; Phillips et al. 2000; Ulfberg et al. 2001). Unfortunately, only some used the most recent diagnostic criteria; the number of diagnostic questions used to ascertain diagnosis varied from one to four; and only two studies used face-to-face interviews to confirm diagnoses (Nichols et al. 2003; Rothdach et al. 2000). In populations of northern European descent, overall prevalence rates for RLS are roughly 3%–5%, rising roughly linearly with age to a rate of 10%–20% of those over age 65. Lower prevalence rates appear in other ethnic groups, such as Asian (Tan et al. 2001), Turkish (Sevim et al. 2003), and Indian populations (Bhowmik et al. 2003). Regardless of ethnicity, however, women appear to have RLS prevalence rates roughly 50% higher than those of men, and parity may influence prevalence rates (Berger et al. 2004). The majority of individuals with RLS have it on an infrequent basis, roughly 1–4 times per month, and in this way it is more similar to migraine headaches or seizure disorders than to painful conditions such as peripheral neuropathy and osteoarthritis, movement disorders such as Parkinson's disease, or sleep disorders such as sleep apnea, which are present on a daily basis. However, roughly 25% of RLS patients describe symptoms on a daily or near-daily basis.

RLS is more common in individuals with a variety of medical disorders: end-stage renal disease (ESRD) (15%–30%) (Unruh et al. 2004; Winkelman et al. 1996), iron deficiency anemia (Berger et al. 2002), and rheumatoid arthritis (Reynolds et al. 1986). Similarly, it is common in pregnant women, affecting up to 33% of those in the third trimester (Suzuki et al. 2003). In such cases, it is considered to be "secondary" RLS. No consistent phenotypic differences between primary and secondary RLS have been identified, and until proven otherwise, RLS should be considered a syndrome with many underlying etiologies.

RLS can have its onset at any age. In one retrospective review of individuals with RLS, 10%–20% of patients reported having onset of symptoms before age 10, and 40% by age 20 (Walters et al. 1996). A number of studies have demonstrated that those with early onset of RLS (defined variably as before age 30–40) have a much stronger risk of having a family history of RLS (Winkelmann et al. 2000). Children who present with RLS may receive diagnoses of "growing pains" or attention-deficit/hyperactivity disorder (Rajaram et al. 2004). A late onset of RLS suggests that one should search for secondary causes. Although the severity of the disorder has been commonly thought to progress over time, in the absence of good data it is unclear what the course of RLS is once the disorder has become established.

Pathogenesis

At this time, the majority of individuals with RLS must be considered to have idiopathic disease. However, a number of clues to the pathophysiology of the disorder, and some recent exciting scientific findings, suggest that important etiologic discoveries may be close.

A familial aspect to RLS has been recognized for many years; roughly 30%–50% of individuals with RLS report a first-degree family member with the disease (Winkelmann et al. 2000). An autosomal dominant mechanism of inheritance has been suggested by both analysis of single families and a large cosegregation study in individuals with onset before age 30 (Winkelmann et al. 2002). Chromosomal analyses have found significant linkages to chromosome 14q in an Italian family (using an autosomal dominant mechanism) (Bonati et al. 2003); chromosome 12q in a French-Canadian family (dominant mechanism) (Desautels et al. 2001); and chromosome 9p (autosomal dominant mechanism) (Chen et al. 2004). At this point, the belief of researchers in the field is that early-onset RLS has strong genetic influences and that late-onset disease may be more related to secondary causes.

The most prominent etiologic candidate for RLS is an abnormality in the regulation of central nervous system (CNS) iron. Combined with Ekbom's early description of the elevated prevalence of iron deficiency in RLS (Ekbom 1944), newer findings that iron repletion can markedly alleviate symptoms of RLS (in those with iron deficiency) (O'Keeffe et al. 1994) and in those with ESRD (Sloand et al. 2004) have focused attention on the role of iron in the pathophysiology of RLS. Many of the conditions that predispose to secondary RLS, such as pregnancy, rheumatoid arthritis, and ESRD, are associated with iron deficiency. The role of iron in dopamine synthesis and receptor regulation has further reinforced the connection between iron and RLS (Allen 2004). Similarly, iron deficiency is thought to increase the vulnerability to the appearance of akathisia in individuals given typical antipsychotics (Hofmann et al. 2000). A number of studies have confirmed the importance of CNS iron in primary RLS. Ferritin (the protein storage form of iron) in cerebrospinal fluid is low in primary RLS, even when serum iron is normal (Earley et al. 2000); substantia nigra iron levels (measured with T_2-weighted magnetic resonance imaging) are low in RLS (Allen et al. 2001); and iron levels are low in substantia nigra at autopsy in individuals with RLS (Connor et al. 2003). These findings suggest that transport of iron into the CNS or into the cell, and/or utilization of iron intracellularly, may be impaired in RLS.

The successful treatment of RLS with dopaminergic precursors and agonists has also focused attention on the dopaminergic system in RLS. In addition, the similarity of RLS to akathisia suggests that the dopaminergic system may be involved. However, studies attempting to demonstrate abnormalities in dopaminergic function in RLS patients have been negative or inconsistent or have shown only minor differences between RLS patients and control subjects. For instance, in the tuberoinfundibular hormonal system (unlikely to be directly related to RLS etiology), dopamine acts as the inhibitor of prolactin—and RLS patients have normal levels of prolactin, and also of all hypothalamic-pituitary-adrenal–related hormones (Wetter et al. 2002). More saliently, although early positron emission tomography (PET) and single-photon emission computed tomography (SPECT) studies of postsynaptic striatal D_2 dopaminergic receptor density found small reductions in RLS patients compared with control subjects (Ruottinen et al. 2000; Turjanski et al. 1999), two more recent studies failed to replicate these findings using SPECT (Eisensehr et al. 2001; Tribl et al. 2002). Furthermore, in distinction to akathisia, RLS is not exacerbated by the dopaminergic antagonist metoclopramide (Winkelmann et al. 2001).

Thus, the status of the hypodopaminergic hypothesis of RLS is unsettled. Investigators are focusing on the A11 dopaminergic system, which originates in the thalamus and descends to the spinal cord (Ondo et al. 2000) and may be relevant to symptoms observed in RLS. The importance of spinal mechanisms in RLS has been emphasized by abnormal flexor withdrawal responses to tibial nerve stimulation (Bara-Jimenez et al. 2000) as well as by the presence of PLMS in patients with cord transections (de Mello et al. 1996).

The diurnal variation in RLS severity has produced other insights into its pathophysiology. Recently, the role of melatonin in RLS has been suggested by the finding of endogenous melatonin release 2 hours before the onset of nocturnal RLS symptoms (Michaud et al. 2004). In addition, RLS patients showed relative enhanced inhibition of prolactin release to a nocturnal L-dopa challenge (vs. a morning challenge) compared with control subjects who did not have RLS, suggesting supersensitivity of dopamine receptors at night in RLS (Garcia-Borreguerro et al. 2004). This diurnal modulation of dopaminergic activity may explain why neuroimaging studies of RLS, which have all been performed during the daytime, may have produced such inconsistent or negative results.

Differential Diagnosis

Severe cases of RLS can generally be easily identified once its cardinal symptoms are understood, but milder cases and cases with atypical presentations can be more difficult to diagnose. Both the sensory and motor symptoms may give rise to confusion, although the improvement with movement as well as the circadian variation can be extremely helpful in clarifying the diagnosis. The dysesthesia of RLS is most difficult to distinguish from that seen with peripheral neuropathy from a variety of causes (e.g., diabetic, toxic, idiopathic), particularly in cases in which RLS is described as "painful." Given the age distribution of neuropathies and of RLS, these two disorders not uncommonly co-occur, although it does not appear that there is a higher prevalence of RLS in those with neuropathy (Rutkove et al. 1996). Further contributing to the diagnostic difficulties is the observation that painful peripheral neuropathy worsens at night in more than 50% of cases; however, it generally does not improve with movement. On the other hand, nocturnal leg cramps, which do occur at night and do improve with movement, may also be difficult to distinguish from RLS on cursory interview. However, nocturnal leg cramps arise precipitously from sleep and are not associated with a feeling of motor restlessness.

The motor restlessness of RLS is most commonly confused with akathisia, anxiety disorders, or attention-deficit/hyperactivity disorder. Distinguishing between RLS and akathisia can be difficult. With waning prescription of typical antipsychotics, the most common cause of akathisia may be related to serotonergic antidepressants (Lane 1998). A number of small case series and clinical reports have been published describing such akathisias (Gerber and Lynd 1998). However, even with careful reading of these case descriptions it is difficult to distinguish akathisia from medication-related RLS. Similarly, description of a worsening or de novo appearance of RLS with serotonergic antidepressants does not clarify this issue. Because both RLS and serotonergic antidepressant–

related akathisia are clinical diagnoses, and both may produce PLMS (Salin-Pascual et al. 1997), clinical and polysomnographic differentiation is difficult. However, a history of RLS prior to the antidepressant administration, the presence of a sensory component, a nocturnal worsening of symptoms, and a therapeutic response to dopaminergic agonists all suggest a diagnosis of RLS. Anxiety associated with bedtime and sleep onset can manifest with inability to get comfortable, restlessness, and vague sensory complaints (Perlis et al. 1997). However, a lack of localization to the legs, the strict localization of the experience to the bed, and the presence of anxiety regarding sleeplessness all suggest a diagnosis of conditioned or psychophysiological insomnia rather than RLS.

The habitual behaviors of feet rubbing or body rocking, called rhythmic movement disorders, may also mimic RLS. In fact, these behaviors may have similar etiologies to RLS, and until the pathophysiology of all these disorders is better understood, a final opinion on their relationship must be reserved (Lombardi et al. 2003). Some rare neurologic disorders may also mimic RLS, including that of painful toes and moving feet (Dressler et al. 1994).

In the end, given the remarkable effectiveness of treatments for RLS and their relative lack of substantial side effects, an empiric course of treatment appears indicated when there is a high enough index of suspicion that RLS may be present. Although treatment success at these times does not clinch a diagnosis of RLS, very few other disorders that are in the differential diagnosis of RLS respond to dopaminergic agonists.

Treatment

Treatments for RLS have evolved substantially since the 1980s. Currently, clinical algorithms (Earley 2003; Silber et al. 2004) recommend that treatment be initially directed towards reversible causes (secondary RLS) such as iron deficiency, antidepressant-related RLS, or opiate withdrawal. If underlying causes of RLS cannot be identified or (as in ESRD) cannot be modified, treatments of primary and of secondary RLS are nearly identical (see Figure 5–4). In addition to the use of specific medications for RLS, a number of behavioral issues are relevant. Both caffeine and alcohol can exacerbate RLS, and their use within 12 hours of bedtime should be avoided. RLS is (by definition) worse with immobility, and individuals should avoid unnecessary immobility, thereby limiting the period of time for which RLS symptoms require treatment. In addition, individuals with RLS are encouraged to aim for 80%–90% (rather than 100%) control of symptoms outside of the sleep setting because this strategy will limit the dose and duration of treatment. In individuals who have symptoms on a non-nightly basis, medications may be used on an as-needed basis. Sleep deprivation should be avoided because it also appears to aggravate RLS symptoms.

Historically, Sir Thomas Willis recommended treatment with laudanum, an opium derivative (Winkelmann 1999). In the 1970s and 1980s, RLS (if treated) was treated with benzodiazepines, similarly to other insomnias. Subsequently, however, the special value of dopaminergic agents in the treatment of RLS was demonstrated, and they are now considered first-line treatments, although few head-to-head trials of these agents versus other alternatives (opiates, anticonvulsants, benzodiazepines) are available. It should be emphasized that dopaminergic agonists can exacerbate underlying psychosis, and thus these medications should be administered with extreme caution in patients with a psychotic disorder.

The value of L-dopa for RLS was first demonstrated in the 1980s (Akpinar 1982). L-dopa provided the first relief for many people who had endured many years of substantial suffering with RLS. Studies using L-dopa demonstrated dramatic improvements in RLS symptoms in the evening and a shortening of latency to sleep onset (Trenkwalder et al. 1995). Because of the short period during which L-dopa enhances central dopaminergic transmission, some studies found a "rebound" of RLS symptoms in the second half of the night and in the morning. For this reason, a combination of short- and long-acting L-dopa was commonly used, with improved clinical results (Collado-Seidel et al. 1999). The dramatic effectiveness of L-dopa not only transformed the clinical approach to RLS, but created a rationale for the study of RLS pathophysiology, the dopaminergic hypothesis (discussed above under "Pathogenesis").

Moderate to severe daily RLS

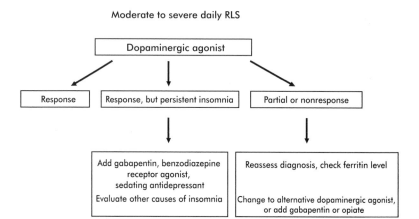

Figure 5–4. Algorithm for the treatment of restless legs syndrome (RLS).

Although L-dopa treatment is extremely effective for RLS symptoms, two complications have led to its decline as a first-line therapy: augmentation and tolerance. Augmentation is the progressively earlier appearance of RLS symptoms during the day during chronic therapy, and it is observed in roughly two-thirds of individuals treated with L-dopa for RLS (Allen and Earley 1996). For instance, in a patient who originally describes symptom onset at 10:00 P.M., L-dopa use over a period of months might lead to earlier and earlier symptoms, such that restlessness or dysesthesia might begin at 4:00–6:00 P.M., or even in the morning. Unfortunately, treatment earlier in the day with L-dopa only exacerbates this complication, and some individuals may end up with round-the-clock severe symptomatology. Other aspects of augmentation, less frequently encountered, include an extension of RLS symptoms to other body parts than the legs (in particular, to the arms), a shorter duration of treatment effectiveness after medication administration, and a shorter period of immobility before RLS symptoms occur. Tolerance to L-dopa is manifested by a reduced effectiveness of the medication over time in the alleviation of RLS symptoms (Allen and Earley 1996).

In response to these complications of L-dopa treatment, longer-acting dopaminergic agonists have become the standard first-line therapy for RLS, in the belief that half-life may be an important predictor of augmentation. A number of these agents are available (see Table 5–2); all have U.S. Food and Drug Administration approval for the treatment of Parkinson's disease, and some should have a specific RLS indication in the near future. The most commonly used medications in this group are pramipexole, ropinirole, and pergolide. The binding profiles of these dopaminergic agonists to the subtypes of dopaminergic receptors (D_1–D_5) remains in dispute; however, it appears that pramipexole has a higher affinity for the dopamine D_3 receptor than does ropinirole (Piercey 1998). The importance of this distinction for the treatment of RLS is unclear, although the prevalence of D_3 receptors in the limbic system might have some importance for psychiatric influences of these medications (Goldberg et al. 2004).

Pramipexole's effectiveness in RLS was demonstrated in a small study of 10 patients with severe RLS, in which striking improvements in both RLS symptoms and periodic limb movement index were observed at 1.5 mg/day (Montplaisir et al. 1999). A larger case series of RLS patients treated with pramipexole found that more than 90% obtained at least partial relief of RLS with the medication (Silber et al. 2003). Two long-term naturalistic follow-up studies of pramipexole both found that one-third of patients taking this agent developed augmentation, with the mean occurrence appearing 8–12 months after initiation of treatment (Silber et al. 2003; Winkelman and Johnston 2004). In general, augmentation with pramipexole was nearly always managed by somewhat earlier dosing of medication (e.g., 6:00 P.M.), and the severe augmentation observed with L-dopa was only rarely observed in these case series.

The most extensive research using a dopaminergic agonist in RLS has been performed with ropinirole, in which two double-blind, placebo-controlled, randomized studies have shown benefit of this agent for both RLS and PLMS, using average doses of 2 mg before bedtime (Adler et al. 2004; Trenkwalder et al. 2004a). Long-term studies of ropinirole are not currently available. Two double-blind, placebo-controlled studies have been published using pergolide for the treatment of RLS, again showing significant benefit compared with placebo (Trenkwalder et al. 2004b; Wetter et al. 1999).

Table 5–2. Commonly used medications for the treatment of restless legs syndrome

Medication	Starting dose (mg)	Target dose (mg)	Administration	Common side effects
Dopamine agents				
Levodopa/carbidopa (Sinemet)	25/100	50/200	1 hour before symptoms onset or q 4–6 h	Nausea, headache
Pergolide (Permax)	0.05	0.20–0.50	2 hours before symptom onset or 6:00 P.M.	Nausea, nasal stuffiness
Pramipexole (Mirapex)	0.125–0.25	0.25–0.75	2 hours before symptom onset; may require 6:00 P.M. and qhs	Fatigue, insomnia, nausea, headache
Ropinirole (Requip)	0.25	1.5–4.0	2 hours before symptom onset; may require 6:00 P.M. and qhs	Nausea, fatigue, headache
Anticonvulsants				
Gabapentin (Neurontin)	100–300	600–1,200	qhs or 6:00 P.M. and qhs	Sedation, ataxia
Opioids				
Codeine (Tylenol #3)	300/30	30–60	1 hour before symptom onset or q 4–6 h	Sedation, insomnia, dry mouth, constipation
Oxycodone (Percocet)	5	5–15	1 hour before symptom onset or q 4–6 h	Sedation, insomnia, dry mouth, constipation
Benzodiazepines				
Clonazepam (Klonopin)	0.5	0.5	1 hour before symptom onset or qhs	Sedation, ataxia, memory impairment
Lorazepam (Ativan)	1	1–2	1 hour before symptom onset or qhs	Sedation, ataxia, memory impairment

No randomized, blinded studies have been performed comparing different dopaminergic agents. In general, pramipexole and ropinirole are more commonly used than pergolide for the treatment of RLS because pergolide's side effect profile, particularly nausea and severe nasal stuffiness, is associated with substantial tolerability issues. Furthermore, pleuropulmonary fibrosis and valvular heart defects, which are rare complications of such ergot-derived medications, have been observed with this agent (Danoff et al. 2001). On the other hand, the profiles of pramipexole and ropinirole are very similar. The former has a somewhat longer half-life (8 hours vs. 6 hours), which may produce therapeutic benefit throughout the evening and night with a single 6:00 P.M. dose. On the other hand, ropinirole has a shorter T_{max} (time to maximum plasma concentration) and thus may provide faster relief of symptoms.

The majority of postmarketing data suggests that most individuals with RLS obtain substantial relief of the core RLS symptoms with dopaminergic therapies. However, more severely afflicted individuals may continue to be only partially responsive to monotherapy (usually with a dopaminergic agent). In these cases, additional treatment with an adjunctive agent is indicated. The best second-line agents for RLS, and thus the most effective add-on agents, are the opiates and gabapentin. Oxycodone and codeine are the most commonly used medications in this class (Walters et al. 2001). The choice of opiate agent is usually based on the duration of action required, which depends on the time of initial onset of refractory symptoms. Most commonly, symptoms that respond only partially to dopaminergic agents occur before bedtime or during nocturnal awakenings, and thus oxycodone or codeine is generally effective, usually in low doses. In more severely affected individuals, who may report refractory distressing symptoms throughout the day, use of long-acting oxycodone, morphine, or methadone may be necessary. Of course, caution should always be practiced when prescribing opiates, given their potential for abuse and respiratory suppression.

Anticonvulsants may also be of therapeutic value for RLS in cases where a dopaminergic agonist produces only partial response, is not well tolerated, or is contraindicated. Controlled trials demonstrated a significant advantage of both gabapentin (Garcia-Borreguerro et al. 2002) and carbamazepine (Telstad et al. 1984) compared with placebo. Gabapentin is not as effective in reducing PLMS as dopaminergic agonists, but, because of its mild sedative effect, it is used as adjunctive treatment in individuals who have persistent sleep disturbance after partial control of RLS symptoms. Similarly, short- to intermediate-acting benzodiazepines can be of value for both mild RLS and persistent sleep disturbance in RLS (Silber et al. 2004). Long-acting benzodiazepines (Saletu et al. 2001) should be reserved for patients with comorbid daytime anxiety disorders, due to the risks of motor incoordination and memory impairment with these longer-acting agents.

Although the dopaminergic agonists are extremely effective for the sensory and motor symptoms of RLS, many treatment studies have demonstrated only modest improvements in sleep efficiency. These findings are reinforced by recent naturalistic data revealing that 33%–60% of patients taking pramipexole for RLS are also taking hypnotics such as benzodiazepines, sedating antidepressants, or anticonvulsants to assist with sleep (Silber et al. 2003; Winkelman and Johnston 2004). The multiple potential causes of persistent poor sleep in individuals with at least partially resolved RLS include refractory RLS or PLMS, conditioned insomnia from long-standing difficulty with sleep, another primary sleep disorder (e.g., sleep apnea), and insomnia related to the RLS medication. It should be recognized that dopaminergic agents may be themselves disruptive to sleep, and that it is primarily their ability to improve the underlying RLS that makes them effective for sleep. In this respect, they are similar to serotonergic treatments for depressive disorders.

Summary

RLS is a common disorder, particularly in older adults, although it is frequently undiagnosed or inadequately treated. A number of developments are driving the field at this time, including increased physician and lay awareness, advances in understanding the pathophysiology of RLS, and rigorous evaluation of a variety of effective treatments.

References

Adler CH, Hauser RA, Sethi K, et al: Ropinirole for restless legs syndrome: a placebo-controlled crossover trial. Neurology 62:1405–1407, 2004

Akpinar S: Treatment of restless legs syndrome with levodopa plus benserazide (letter). Arch Neurol 39:739, 1982

Allen R: Dopamine and iron in the pathophysiology of restless legs syndrome (RLS). Sleep Med 5:385–391, 2004

Allen RP, Earley CJ: Augmentation of the restless legs syndrome with carbidopa/levodopa. Sleep 19:205–213, 1996

Allen RP, Barker PB, Wehrl F, et al: MRI measurement of brain iron in patients with restless legs syndrome. Neurology 56:263–265, 2001

Allen RP, Picchietti D, Hening WA, et al: Restless legs syndrome: diagnostic criteria, special considerations, and epidemiology. A report from the restless legs syndrome diagnosis and epidemiology workshop at the National Institutes of Health. Restless Legs Syndrome Diagnosis and Epidemiology Workshop at the National Institutes of Health; International Restless Legs Syndrome Study Group. Sleep Med 4:101–119, 2003

American Psychiatric Association: Diagnostic and Statistical Manual of Mental Disorders, 4th Edition, Text Revision. Washington, DC, American Psychiatric Association, 2000

Bara-Jimenez W, Aksu M, Graham B, et al: Periodic limb movements in sleep: state-dependent excitability of the spinal flexor reflex. Neurology 54:1609–1616, 2000

Berger K, von Eckardstein A, Trenkwalder C, et al: Iron metabolism and the risk of restless legs syndrome in an elderly general population: the MEMO-Study. J Neurol 249:1195–1199, 2002

Berger K, Luedemann J, Trenkwalder C, et al: Sex and the risk of restless legs syndrome in the general population. Arch Intern Med 164:196–202, 2004

Bhowmik D, Bhatia M, Gupta S, et al: Restless legs syndrome in hemodialysis patients in India: a case controlled study. Sleep Med 4:143–146, 2003

Bonati MT, Ferini-Strambi L, Aridon P, et al: Autosomal dominant restless legs syndrome maps on chromosome 14q. Brain 126:1485–1492, 2003

Chen S, Ondo WG, Rao S, et al: Genomewide linkage scan identifies a novel susceptibility locus for restless legs syndrome on chromosome 9p. Am J Hum Genet 7:876–885, 2004

Collado-Seidel V, Kazenwadel J, Wetter TC, et al: A controlled study of additional sr- L-dopa in L-dopa-responsive restless legs syndrome with late-night symptoms. Neurology 52:285–290, 1999

Connor JR, Boyer PJ, Menzies SL, et al: Neuropathological examination suggests impaired brain iron acquisition in restless legs syndrome. Neurology 61:304–309, 2003

Czeisler CA, Winkelman JW, Richardson GS: Sleep disorders, in Harrison's Principles of Internal Medicine, 16th Edition. Edited by Kasper DL, Braunwald E, Fauci A, et al. New York, McGraw-Hill Professional, 2004, pp 153–162

Danoff SK, Grasso ME, Terry PB, et al: Pleuropulmonary disease due to pergolide use for restless legs syndrome. Chest 120:313–316, 2001

De Mello MT, Lauro FA, Silva AC, et al: Incidence of periodic leg movements and of the restless legs syndrome during sleep following acute physical activity in spinal cord injury subjects. Spinal Cord 34:294–296, 1996

Desautels A, Turecki G, Montplaisir J, et al: Identification of a major susceptibility locus for restless legs syndrome on chromosome 12q. Am J Hum Genet 69:1266–1270, 2001

Dressler D, Thompson PD, Gledhill RF, et al: The syndrome of painful legs and moving toes. Mov Disord 9:13–21, 1994

Earley CJ: Clinical practice: restless legs syndrome. N Engl J Med 348:2103–2109, 2003

Earley CJ, Connor JR, Beard JL, et al: Abnormalities in CSF concentrations of ferritin and transferrin in restless legs syndrome. Neurology 54:1698–1700, 2000

Eisensehr I, Wetter TC, Linke R, et al: Normal IPT and IBZM SPECT in drug-naive and levodopa-treated idiopathic restless legs syndrome. Neurology 57:1307–1309, 2001

Ekbom KA: Asthenia crurum paraesthetica ("Irritable Legs"). Acta Med Scand 118:197–209, 1944

Garcia-Borreguero D, Larrosa O, de la Llave Y, et al: Treatment of restless legs syndrome with gabapentin: a double-blind, cross-over study. Neurology 59:1573–1579, 2002

Garcia-Borreguero D, Larrosa O, Granizo JJ, et al: Circadian variation in neuroendocrine response to L-dopa in patients with restless legs syndrome. Sleep 27:669–673, 2004

Gerber PE, Lynd LD: Selective serotonin-reuptake inhibitor-induced movement disorders. Ann Pharmacother 32:692–698, 1998

Goldberg JF, Burdick KE, Endick CJ: Preliminary randomized, double-blind, placebo-controlled trial of pramipexole added to mood stabilizers for treatment-resistant bipolar depression. Am J Psychiatry 161:564–566, 2004

Hening W, Walters AS, Allen RP, et al: Impact, diagnosis and treatment of restless legs syndrome (RLS) in a primary care population: the REST (RLS Epidemiology, Symptoms, and Treatment) primary care study. Sleep Med 5:237–246, 2004

Hofmann M, Seifritz E, Botschev C, et al: Serum iron and ferritin in acute neuroleptic akathisia. Psychiatry Res 93:201–207, 2000

Lane RM: SSRI-induced extrapyramidal side-effects and akathisia: implications for treatment. J Psychopharmacol 12:192–214, 1998

Lombardi C, Provini F, Vetrugno R, et al: Pelvic movements as rhythmic motor manifestation associated with restless legs syndrome. Mov Disord 18:110–113, 2003

Michaud M, Lavigne G, Desautels A, et al: Effects of immobility on sensory and motor symptoms of restless legs syndrome. Mov Disord 17:112–115, 2002a

Michaud M, Paquet J, Lavigne G, et al: Sleep laboratory diagnosis of restless legs syndrome. Eur Neurol 48:108–113, 2002b

Michaud M, Dumont M, Selmaoui B, et al: Circadian rhythm of restless legs syndrome: relationship with biological markers. Ann Neurol 55:372–380, 2004

Montplaisir J, Nicolas A, Denesle R, et al: Restless legs syndrome improved by pramipexole: a double-blind randomized trial. Neurology 52:938–943, 1999

Montplaisir J, Michaud M, Denesle R, et al: Periodic leg movements are not more prevalent in insomnia or hypersomnia but are specifically associated with sleep disorders involving a dopaminergic impairment. Sleep Med 1:163–167, 2000

Nichols DA, Allen RP, Grauke JH, et al: Restless legs syndrome symptoms in primary care: a prevalence study. Arch Intern Med 163:2323–2329, 2003

Ohayon MM, Roth T: Prevalence of restless legs syndrome and periodic limb movement disorder in the general population. J Psychosom Res 53:547–554, 2002

O'Keeffe ST, Gavin K, Lavan JN: Iron status and restless legs syndrome in the elderly. Age Ageing 23:200–203, 1994

Ondo WG, He Y, Rajasekaran S, et al: Clinical correlates of 6-hydroxydopamine injections into A11 dopaminergic neurons in rats: a possible model for restless legs syndrome. Mov Disord 15:154–158, 2000

Perlis ML, Giles DE, Mendelson WB, et al: Psychophysiological insomnia: the behavioural model and a neurocognitive perspective. J Sleep Res 6:179–188, 1997

Phillips B, Young T, Finn L, et al: Epidemiology of restless legs symptoms in adults. Arch Intern Med 160:2137–2141, 2000

Piercey MF: Pharmacology of pramipexole, a dopamine D_3-preferring agonist useful in treating Parkinson's disease. Clin Neuropharmacol 21:141–151, 1998

Rajaram SS, Walters AS, England SJ, et al: Some children with growing pains may actually have restless legs syndrome. Sleep 27:767–773, 2004

Reynolds G, Blake DR, Pall HS, et al: Restless leg syndrome and rheumatoid arthritis. Br Med J (Clin Res Ed) 292:659–660, 1986

Rothdach AJ, Trenkwalder C, Haberstock J, et al: Prevalence and risk factors of RLS in an elderly population: the MEMO study. Memory and Morbidity in Augsburg Elderly. Neurology 54:1064–1068, 2000

Rutkove SB, Matheson JK, Logigian EL: Restless legs syndrome in patients with polyneuropathy. Muscle Nerve 19:670–672, 1996

Ruottinen HM, Partinen M, Hublin C, et al: An FDOPA PET study in patients with periodic limb movement disorder and restless legs syndrome. Neurology 54:502–504, 2000

Saletu M, Anderer P, Saletu-Zyhlarz G, et al: Restless legs syndrome (RLS) and periodic limb movement disorder (PLMD): acute placebo-controlled sleep laboratory studies with clonazepam. Eur Neuropsychopharmacol 11:153–161, 2001

Salin-Pascual RJ, Galicia-Polo L, Drucker-Colin R: Sleep changes after 4 consecutive days of venlafaxine administration in normal volunteers. J Clin Psychiatry 58:348–350, 1997

Sevim S, Dogu O, Camdeviren H, et al: Unexpectedly low prevalence and unusual characteristics of RLS in Mersin, Turkey. Neurology 61:1562–1569, 2003

Silber MH, Girish M, Izurieta R: Pramipexole in the management of restless legs syndrome: an extended study. Sleep 26:819–821, 2003

Silber MH, Ehrenberg BL, Allen RP, et al: An algorithm for the management of restless legs syndrome. Medical Advisory Board of the Restless Legs Syndrome Foundation. Mayo Clin Proc 79:916–922, 2004

Sloand JA, Shelly MA, Feigin A, et al: A double-blind, placebo-controlled trial of intravenous iron dextran therapy in patients with ESRD and restless legs syndrome. Am J Kidney Dis 43:663–670, 2004

Suzuki K, Ohida T, Sone T, et al: The prevalence of restless legs syndrome among pregnant women in Japan and the relationship between restless legs syndrome and sleep problems. Sleep 26:673–677, 2003

Tan EK, Seah A, See SJ, et al: Restless legs syndrome in an Asian population: a study in Singapore. Mov Disord 16:577–579, 2001

Telstad W, Sorensen O, Larsen S, et al: Treatment of the restless legs syndrome with carbamazepine: a double blind study. Br Med J (Clin Res Ed) 288:444–446, 1984

Trenkwalder C, Stiasny K, Pollmacher T, et al: L-Dopa therapy of uremic and idiopathic restless legs syndrome: a double-blind, crossover trial. Sleep 18:681–688, 1995

Trenkwalder C, Garcia-Borreguero D, Montagna P, et al: Ropinirole in the treatment of restless legs syndrome: results from the TREAT RLS 1 study, a 12 week, randomised, placebo controlled study in 10 European countries. Therapy With Ropinirole; Efficacy and Tolerability in RLS 1 Study Group. J Neurol Neurosurg Psychiatry 75:92–97, 2004a

Trenkwalder C, Hundemer HP, Lledo A, et al: Efficacy of pergolide in treatment of restless legs syndrome: the PEARLS Study. PEARLS Study Group. Neurology 62:1391–1397, 2004b

Tribl GG, Asenbaum S, Klosch G, et al: Normal IPT and IBZM SPECT in drug naive and levodopa-treated idiopathic restless legs syndrome. Neurology 59:649–650, 2002

Turjanski N, Lees AJ, Brooks DJ: Striatal dopaminergic function in restless legs syndrome: 18F-dopa and 11C-raclopride PET studies. Neurology 52:932–937, 1999

Ulfberg J, Nystrom B, Carter N, et al: Prevalence of restless legs syndrome among men aged 18 to 64 years: an association with somatic disease and neuropsychiatric symptoms. Mov Disord 16:1159–1163, 2001

Unruh ML, Levey AS, D'Ambrosio C, et al: Restless legs symptoms among incident dialysis patients: association with lower quality of life and shorter survival. Choices for Healthy Outcomes in Caring for End-Stage Renal Disease (CHOICE) Study. Am J Kidney Dis 43:900–909, 2004

Walters AS: Toward a better definition of the restless legs syndrome. The International Restless Legs Syndrome Study Group. Mov Disord 10:634–642, 1995

Walters AS, Hickey K, Maltzman J, et al: A questionnaire study of 138 patients with restless legs syndrome: the "Night-Walkers" survey. Neurology 46:92–95, 1996

Walters AS, Winkelmann J, Trenkwalder C, et al: Long-term follow-up on restless legs syndrome patients treated with opioids. Mov Disord 16:1105–1109, 2001

Wetter TC, Stiasny K, Winkelmann J, et al: A randomized controlled study of pergolide in patients with restless legs syndrome. Neurology 52:944–950, 1999

Wetter TC, Collado-Seidel V, Oertel H, et al: Endocrine rhythms in patients with restless legs syndrome. J Neurol 249:146–151, 2002

Winkelman JW: The evoked heart rate response to periodic leg movements of sleep. Sleep 22:575–580, 1999

Winkelman JW, Johnston L: Augmentation and tolerance with long-term pramipexole treatment of restless legs syndrome (RLS). Sleep Med 5:9–14, 2004

Winkelman JW, Chertow GM, Lazarus JM: Restless legs syndrome in end-stage renal disease. Am J Kidney Dis 28:372–378, 1996

Winkelmann J: Restless legs syndrome. Arch Neurol 56:1526–1527, 1999

Winkelmann J, Wetter TC, Collado-Seidel V, et al: Clinical characteristics and frequency of the hereditary restless legs syndrome in a population of 300 patients. Sleep 23:597–600, 2000

Winkelmann J, Schadrack J, Wetter TC, et al: Opioid and dopamine antagonist drug challenges in untreated restless legs syndrome patients. Sleep Med 2:57–61, 2001

Winkelmann J, Muller-Myhsok B, Wittchen HU, et al: Complex segregation analysis of restless legs syndrome provides evidence for an autosomal dominant mode of inheritance in early age at onset families. Ann Neurol 52:297–302, 2002

Chapter 6

Parasomnias

John W. Winkelman, M.D., Ph.D.

The class of sleep disorders known as parasomnias comprises some of the most unusual, challenging and potentially instructive of all behavioral disorders. The term *parasomnia* derives from the Latin "para" meaning next to, and "somnus" referring to sleep. In the proposed *International Classification of Sleep Disorders*, 2nd Edition (American Academy of Sleep Medicine, in press), parasomnias are defined as "undesirable physical or experiential events that accompany sleep." It is this admixture of the sleeping mind and apparently purposeful behavior that not only challenges our definitions and understanding of willed behavior, but can also teach us about the characteristics of rapid eye movement (REM) and non–rapid eye movement (non-REM) sleep and their interactions with wakefulness.

Parasomnias are generally divided into those arising from non-REM sleep and those occurring during REM sleep (Table 6–1). Because of the distinctive characteristics of these two sleep states, these two types of parasomnias can often be distinguished by the time of night occurrence, type of mentation during the event, mental status on awakening, duration, degree of amnesia for the event, and associated autonomic activation. Thus, with a few simple questions, parasomnias can often be correctly classified by the clinician.

Non-REM Parasomnias

Our understanding of non-REM parasomnias is based on the concept that arousal from sleep is not an all-or-none phenomenon, but rather a continuum of reestablishment of full alertness, judgment, and control over behavior, and/or a rapid alternation of sleep and waking states (Mahowald and Schenck 2001). Thus, behaviors or mood states can be expressed during such partial arousals, which then are at least partially divorced from full awareness both during the event and on awakening. Most commonly, such behaviors are dissociated motor activities (walking, eating, sexual behavior) or emotional responses (fear, anger, sexual excitement) (Schenck and Mahowald 2000b). They are distinct from waking behavior in that complex mentation is usually not present, feedback from the environment is usually given less salience, and sound judgment is usually not present. It is unclear to what extent these behaviors or emotional states are related to waking motivation, psychological state, or psychopathology. It is clear that these behaviors run in families (Mahowald 2004).

The non-REM parasomnias share many features that may eventually provide insight into their pathophysiology. They are commonly brief, are more frequently expressed in children, are associated with amnesia, and occur in the first 1–2 hours of sleep, usually arising from slow-wave sleep. These disorders will be presented here along a continuum of arousal, beginning with confusional arousals and ending with sleep terrors.

Confusional Arousals

Confusional arousals are usually brief, simple motor behaviors and usually occur without substantial affective expression. Mental confusion, automatic behavior, indistinct speech, and relative unresponsiveness to the environment are hallmarks of a confusional arousal (Ohayon et al. 1999). Sitting up in bed with simple vocalization or picking at bedclothes are common examples. Such behaviors are brief, and amnesia for them is so dense that without a bedpartner's or parent's report, they might go unnoticed. For this reason, epidemiologic information is unreliable. Nevertheless, roughly 10%–20% of children and 2%–5% of adults report a history of confusional arousals (Ohayon et al. 1999). As in all non-REM parasomnias, the expression of confusional arousals appears to depend on a genetic predisposition combined with a precipitating event, which may be endogenous (e.g., a respiratory obstructive event, pain, or leg movement of sleep)

Table 6–1. Overview of parasomnias

Characteristic	Non-REM parasomnias				REM-related parasomnias	
	Confusional arousals	Sleepwalking	Sleep terrors	SRED	RBD	Nightmare disorder
Stage of arousal	II, III, IV	III, IV	III, IV	II, III, IV	REM	REM
Time of night	Anytime	First 2 hours	First 2 hours	Anytime	Anytime	Anytime
EEG profile with event	NA	Mixed	Mixed	Mixed	Characteristic of REM	NA
EMG activity with event	High	High	High	High	High, variable	NA
Relative unresponsiveness during event	Yes	Yes	Yes	Yes	Yes	Yes
Autonomic activity	Low	Low	High	Low	High	High
Amnesia	Yes	Yes	Yes	Partial	No	No
Confusion following episode	Yes	Yes	Yes	Yes	No	No
Family history of parasomnias	Yes	Yes	Yes	Yes	No	No

Note. REM=rapid eye movement; EEG=electroencephalogram; EMG=electromyogram; NA=not available; RBD= REM sleep behavior disorder.

or exogenous (e.g., forced awakening or environmental disruption) (Hublin et al. 2001; Laberge et al. 2000). In predisposed individuals, sleep deprivation, medications, sleep disorders, stress, and circadian misalignment may all aggravate or expose this underlying parasomnia. It is unclear why such partial arousals are more common in children.

Confusional arousals usually arise within the first part of the sleep episode, most commonly during slow-wave sleep. Electroencephalographic recording (EEG) at the time of the episode may show delta waves (characteristic of slow-wave sleep), theta or alpha activity, or alternation between sleep and waking activity (Gaudreau et al. 2000). Confusional arousals may also occur from daytime naps. Individuals do not report dreams on achieving full alertness, but rather an absence of mentation.

Variants of confusional arousals have been recently identified in adults: excessive sleep inertia ("sleep drunkenness") (Roth et al. 1972), abnormal sleep-related sexual behavior ("sexsomnia") (Shapiro et al. 2003), and sleep-related violence (Cartwright 2004). Unlike confusional arousals, *sleep drunkenness* arises from final awakenings in the morning, but in other respects it is similar to events arising from slow-wave sleep, involving slowed mentation, automatic behavior, and relative unresponsiveness to the environment. At such times, individuals may report having substantial difficulty arising or completing even the simplest tasks, and such problems then interfere with daily activities. *Sleep-related abnormal sexual behavior* can include any type of sexual behavior (intercourse, masturbation), but typically it is distinct from the individual's usual behavior in terms of partner (e.g., attempting sexual behavior with a family member) or sexual act (e.g., anal intercourse). Like other confusional arousals, it occurs with limited awareness during the sexual act, relative unresponsiveness to the external environment, and amnesia for the event. *Sleep-related violence* is also generally distinct from the individual's usual behavior. It occurs in a state consistent with night terrors, with anger or fear as the dominant emotion, agitated resistance to the environment, a slow return to normal levels of alertness following the event, and subsequent amnesia for the behavior. The majority of reported cases have been young to middle-aged males with a prior history of sleepwalking

(Bonkalo 1974). Sleep-related sexual and violent behaviors have been the subject of recent medicolegal proceedings, and therefore there is a sense of urgency in establishing a more comprehensive scientific and clinical evidence basis for these parasomnias.

Sleepwalking

Sleepwalking, although it involves more elaborate behavior than simple confusional arousals, forms a continuum with them. It usually occurs within the first hour or two of sleep, often without substantial affective activity. Simple motivations are usually pursued, such as attempts to use the bathroom, go to the kitchen, or, in some cases, leave the home. Although the walker's eyes are open, behavior may be clumsy (Crisp 1996; Kavey et al. 1990). Dreaming is usually not present, and individuals if awakened will report only simple mentation (e.g., "had to find my ring"). Similarly, if sleepwalking is interrupted by family members, responses may be absent, incomplete, or inappropriate, although it is unclear whether this is due to abnormalities in input or output channels. If left alone, sleepwalkers will usually return to sleep, at times in unusual places, but if aroused by family members or as a result of their inappropriate behavior, they may take a long time to come to full awareness. At times, individuals may be violent or agitated if sleepwalking episodes are interrupted. As in other non-REM parasomnias, full or partial amnesia is usually present for the episode.

Sleepwalking occurs in 10%–20% of children and 1%–4% of adults (Laberge et al. 2000; Ohayon et al. 1999). It is most common in children between 5 and 10 years old and becomes less and less prevalent with increasing age. There do not appear to be gender or racial differences in prevalence rates of sleepwalking. Genetic factors appear to play an important role in sleepwalking, as evidenced by both epidemiologic studies and those of twins (Hublin et al. 1997, 2001). Risk of sleepwalking roughly doubles with one parent with a sleepwalking history and triples when both parents have such a history. The variance attributed to genetic factors for sleepwalking is thought to be 60%–80%.

Roughly 80% of adults with sleepwalking have it as a continuation of a childhood behavior, although many of these individuals will not come to medical attention until their twenties or thirties, when they begin to cohabit and the behavior becomes recognized, bothersome, or of concern to the bedpartner. The frequency of sleepwalking has a wide range, although it is uncommon to exhibit the behavior nightly, or even weekly. However, it is the individuals with more frequent sleepwalking who most often come to medical attention.

The relationship between psychiatric disorders and sleepwalking has been controversial (Schenck and Mahowald 2000a). Although childhood sleepwalking does not appear to be associated with psychiatric disorder, a variety of psychiatric disorders may increase the risk of persistence of sleepwalking into adulthood (Gau and Soong 1999; Ohayon et al. 1999). However, it is not believed that sleepwalking represents latent psychopathology or that sleepwalking behaviors are a manifestation of underlying "true" motivations of the sufferer (Hartman et al. 2001). That being said, psychiatric medications may raise the risk of sleepwalking because of their sleep-disruptive or sleep-enhancing properties (Landry et al. 1999). Similarly, stress, sleep deprivation (Joncas et al. 2002), and chaotic sleep schedules may increase the risk of sleepwalking, and each of these precipitants may be more common in the psychiatric patient.

Attempts to document sleepwalking in a sleep laboratory are usually frustrating. It has long been noted that even individuals with nightly sleepwalking do not exhibit the behavior when being monitored (Broughton 1968). For this reason, markers of sleepwalking susceptibility have been investigated as a source of both pathophysiologic and diagnostic information. Most, but not all, polysomnographic studies of sleepwalkers have demonstrated an increase in brief arousals from slow-wave sleep, with preservation of a sleeping EEG accompanied by autonomic activation (increased heart rate and respiration) following the arousal (Espa et al. 2000; Gaudreau et al. 2000). Sleep studies are often performed in such patients (particularly in an adult with a new onset of sleepwalking) to determine whether there is an identifiable precipitant to the inappropriate slow-wave arousal, such as a sleep-related breathing disorder, periodic limb movements of sleep (PLMS), or nocturnal seizures.

Sleep Terrors

Sleep terrors have many of the properties of somnambulism, but they are characterized by more intense motor and autonomic activity and are distinguished by the intensity of the affective expression and experience. Rather than construing them as absolutely distinctive disorders, it is probably more appropriate to consider sleepwalking and sleep terrors as related behaviors that can, in fact, evolve from one to the other during an episode. In children, sleep terrors are classically heralded by a piercing scream, with obvious extreme fear, crying, and inconsolability (Mehlenbeck et al. 2000). In adults, agitation is common, frequently involving the belief that there is an imminent threat and a need for escape or defense (Schenck et al. 1997). For this reason, sleep terror sufferers may cause injury to themselves, to others, or to property in their highly motivated but often clumsy fervor. As in sleepwalking, dreaming is usually not reported, but simple thoughts are present (e.g., "the room is on fire" or "I am being attacked") and can be difficult to dispel even after the person has awakened. If interfered with, a person with a sleep terror may incorporate the other person into the threatening scenario, potentially harming him or her. For this reason, it is recommended that individuals having a sleep terror be gently redirected in an attempt to raise their level of consciousness. As with somnambulism, recollection of the event afterwards is fragmentary, at best.

Sleep terrors are less common than sleepwalking; roughly 5% of children and 1%–2% of adults report a history of such events (Ohayon et al. 1999). As with somnambulism, genetic factors appear to play a role in susceptibility to sleep terrors, and precipitating factors can be either endogenous (e.g., a sleep disorder) or exogenous (an environmental disturbance) (Kales et al. 1980). Arousals usually occur from slow-wave sleep, in the first third of the sleep period. Polysomnography may not capture such an episode, although multiple brief arousals with autonomic hyperactivity from slow-wave sleep may be observed as a marker of the disorder (Llorente et al. 1992).

A number of disorders need to be considered in evaluating patients with episodes of abnormal, unwanted nocturnal motor or affective behaviors. These include nocturnal panic attacks, nocturnal dissociative episodes, frontal lobe seizures, delirium associated with medical or neurologic disorders, and REM sleep behavior disorder. In determining the diagnosis, a daytime history of behaviors similar to the nocturnal behaviors (e.g., panic or dissociative episode) would certainly direct the diagnosis away from a non-REM parasomnia. Similarly, overnight polysomnography might assist in the diagnosis of REM sleep behavior disorder (RBD) or a seizure disorder. Finally, as described above for confusional arousals, elimination of a precipitant of a disordered arousal, whether exogenous (e.g., noise) or endogenous (e.g., sleep apnea, restless legs syndrome, PLMS, nocturia) may prevent the parasomnia from manifesting itself.

Treatment of Non-REM Parasomnias

The decision to treat non-REM parasomnias is based on the frequency of the parasomnia event, the risk of associated injury to self or others, and the distress the behavior is causing the patient or family members (Schenck and Mahowald 2000b). Fortunately, parasomnias occur infrequently for the majority of adult sufferers, but unfortunately, their appearance is unpredictable. Thus, for those individuals with high-risk episodes, the question is whether chronic treatment of episodic events should be chosen.

For most children, parasomnias do not require treatment because there is little or no risk of harm and, although the parents' sleep may be disrupted, the child is unaware of the events both during the night and the following day. Regularization of the sleep-wake cycle and avoidance of sleep deprivation will reduce the frequency of events. For children and young adults who sleepwalk, enhancing the safety of the sleeping environment, such as by locking doors and windows and keeping hallways and stairs well lit, is essential.

When treatment of sleepwalking or sleep terrors in an adult is warranted, a three-step approach is used: modifying predisposing and precipitating factors, enhancing the safety of the sleeping environment, and, if these are not successful, pharmacotherapy. Sleep disorders (e.g., sleep apnea, PLMS), symptoms of medical disorders (pain, nocturia, dyspnea), and medications that are thought to be contributing to sleep instability should be modified to the extent possible. The patient should be kept safe if wandering is an issue. If the parasomnia occurs within the first half of the sleep period, short-acting benzodiazepine receptor agonists such as triazolam (0.125–0.5 mg hs) or zolpidem (5–10 mg hs) are recommended. The most data on treatment of non-REM parasomnias exist for clonazepam (0.5–2.0 mg qhs), which has been used successfully for sleepwalking and sleep terrors for extended periods without the development of tolerance in most patients (Schenck and Mahowald 1996a). It is unclear whether these medications work by suppressing arousals during sleep or by decreasing slow-wave sleep, and no controlled trials have tested their efficacy. However, beneficial clinical experience makes them first-line agents for this purpose (see Table 6–2).

Sleep-Related Eating Disorder

In distinction to the previously discussed non-REM disorders, which have been described for centuries, sleep-related eating disorder (SRED) has only recently come to medical attention, and thus the amount of information regarding its description, course, prevalence, and treatment is more limited. SRED combines features of a sleep disorder (sleepwalking) with those of an eating disorder (binge eating disorder) (Schenck et al. 1991; Winkelman 1998). The behavior consists of repetitive partial arousals from sleep with ingestion of food in a compulsive or driven, often rushed, manner, although individuals with this behavior will later report not having felt hungry at the time they were eating. The chosen foods are typically high in carbohydrates and often are those that the individual would not eat during the daytime. In distinction to the majority of those with sleepwalking, those with SRED will usually engage in this behavior on a nightly basis or multiple times per night. Recollection of the event is usually impaired, and individuals will report that they were half-awake, half-asleep during the eating episode. However, level of awareness may vary across eating episodes within one night as well as across the longitudinal course of SRED over a number of years. Individuals are often very ashamed of the behavior, frequently gain weight as a result of it, and usually alter their daytime consumption of food through morning anorexia and efforts to limit the consumed calories within a 24-hour period.

Preliminary prevalence data suggest that SRED is present in 1%–5% of adults, is 2–4 times more common in females, and most commonly has its onset in late adolescence or early adulthood (Winkelman et al. 1999). It appears to be a chronic disorder, and those seen in a clinical setting have frequently engaged in nocturnal eating for many years before presenting for medical care. SRED appears to be more common in those with a daytime eating disorder (Winkelman et al. 1999), but only a minority of those with SRED have anorexia, bulimia, or daytime binge eating disorder (Schenck et al. 1993). A history of sleepwalking is commonly found in those with SRED, but once nocturnal eating becomes established, other sleepwalking behaviors are usually not observed. Restless legs syndrome is also commonly observed in those with SRED, and treatment of restless legs syndrome can eliminate the nocturnal eating disorder. There is also a suggestion that benzodiazepine receptor agonists can produce SRED (Morgenthaler and Silber 2002). Roughly one-third of individuals with SRED have a first-degree family member with the disorder, consistent with the familial patterns observed in both sleepwalking (Hublin et al. 1997) and certain daytime eating disorders (Klump et al. 2001).

Polysomnographic study has shown that eating episodes in SRED, in distinction to behaviors in the other non-REM parasomnias described above, can occur at any time of the night and from all stages of non-REM sleep (Winkelman 1998). However, polysomnographic features characteristic of sleepwalking (e.g., frequent arousals from slow-wave sleep) are commonly observed (Schenck et al. 1991). The underlying pathophysiology of SRED is unclear. Although abnormalities in the expression of peptides regulating both appetite and the sleep-wake cycle have been described (Birketvedt et al. 1999), it is unclear whether these are a cause or a consequence of the disordered eating and sleep-wake cycle.

The major differential diagnosis is between SRED and nocturnal eating syndrome (NES). NES is a disorder in which the individual eats an excessive amount of food either before bed or during nocturnal awakenings while maintaining full consciousness (Marshall et al. 2004). Sleep disorders are less commonly observed in NES, and a self-report of awareness during the eating episode establishes the diagnosis. However, it should be recognized that level of awareness during nocturnal eating episodes can vary across one night's multiple episodes, as well as across episodes within months or years of nocturnal eating. Thus, NES and SRED should be considered ends of a continuum of related nocturnal eating disorders.

Treatment of SRED is based on the presumed underlying cause of the abnormal arousals and/or disordered eating (see Table 6–2). Individuals with a history of sleepwalking can be administered short- to intermediate-acting benzodiazepines or other non-appetite-stimulating sedatives (e.g., trazodone). However, one complication of this approach has been to aggravate the dissociated eating and amnesia. Alternatively, use of agents that suppress or normalize disordered eating, such as selective serotonin reuptake inhibitors or topiramate (Winkelman 2003), have been effective in some case series. Treatment of patients with SRED (particularly if they have restless legs syndrome) with dopaminergic agonists has proved extremely useful, at times eliminating behaviors that have been present nightly for decades (Schenck et al. 1993). Finally, the safety of the sleeping environment and the avoidance of sleep deprivation and of an irregular sleep schedule are essential, as in treatment of other non-REM parasomnias. In addition, normalization of a daytime eating schedule is important.

REM-Related Parasomnias

REM Sleep Behavior Disorder

Dreaming and paralysis, the distinguishing features of REM sleep, play decisive roles in the expression of RBD by their presence and pathological absence, respectively. In RBD the usual atonia of REM sleep is absent, allowing the sleeper to enact dreams, with potential resulting injury to the sleeper or bedpartner if the behavior is agitated or violent (Schenck and Mahowald 2002). During such episodes, the sleeper's eyes remain closed and he or she is completely unresponsive to the environment until awakened, at which point the person will achieve rapid and

Table 6–2. Pharmacologic treatment of parasomnias

Medication	Effective dose range (mg)	Appropriate patients	Possible side effects
Non-REM parasomnias			
Triazolam	0.125–0.5	First-line treatment	Rebound insomnia on discontinuation
Zolpidem	5–10	Unresponsive to triazolam	Rebound insomnia on discontinuation
Lorazepam	1–2	Unresponsive to shorter-acting agents	Daytime sedation
Clonazepam	0.5–2.0	Unresponsive to shorter-acting agents	Daytime sedation, cognitive dysfunction
Sleep-related eating disorder			
Selective serotonin reuptake inhibitor (e.g., sertraline)	50–200	History of daytime eating, mood, anxiety disorder	Nausea, headache, sexual dysfunction
Topiramate	50–600	Binge eating disorder; insomnia	Paresthesias, cognitive dysfunction
Dopaminergic agonist		Restless legs syndrome (RLS)	Nausea, worsening of RLS
Benzodiazepines		History of sleepwalking	Worsening of amnesia with event, daytime sedation

Table 6–2. Pharmacologic treatment of parasomnias (*continued*)

Medication	Effective dose range (mg)	Appropriate patients	Possible side effects
REM-related parasomnias			
Clonazepam	0.5–2.0	First-line treatment	Daytime sedation, cognitive dysfunction
Lorazepam	1.0–2.0	Side effects with clonazepam	Daytime sedation, cognitive dysfunction
Melatonin	3–15	Unresponsive to benzodiazepines; history of substance abuse	Unknown; daytime sedation
Pramipexole	0.5–1.0	Unresponsive to benzodiazepines; history of substance abuse	Nausea, daytime sedation

full alertness and report a dream that usually corresponds to the exhibited behavior. It is this agitation and/or injury that brings the patient for consultation, usually at the behest of the bedpartner. Episodes of full-blown RBD are intermittent, but it is common for sleeptalking, shouting, or fragmentary motor activity to occur between such events.

RBD is a chronic disorder, usually observed in males above age 50 and in individuals with certain neurologic disorders. In particular, RBD is present in the majority of individuals with neurologic disorders characterized by accumulation of α-synuclein protein (Parkinson's disease, dementia with Lewy bodies, and multiple system atrophy) (Boeve et al. 2003b). In one study, two-thirds of patients with RBD followed for 10 years developed Parkinson's disease, suggesting that the sleep disorder may be an early marker of Parkinson's disease progression (Schenck et al. 1996). Although the site of pathology in RBD is not clear, dopamine transporter abnormalities in the nigrostriatal system have been demonstrated (Eisensehr et al. 2000). Similarly, a reduction in neurons in the peri–locus coeruleus has been seen (Turner et al. 2000). However, more widespread central nervous system dysfunction is suggested by data showing slowing of the EEG during waking as well as subtle neuropsychological dysfunction in patients with idiopathic RBD (Gagnon et al. 2004). An animal model of RBD, in which lesions around the locus coeruleus produced "REM sleep without atonia," was developed well before the description of RBD and implicates these brainstem areas in the control of motor activity in REM sleep (Hendricks et al. 1981).

An important risk factor for RBD of which the psychiatrist should be aware is the use of REM-suppressing antidepressants (serotonergic reuptake inhibitors and monoamine oxidase inhibitors [MAOIs]). Numerous case studies demonstrating appearance of RBD with these agents have been published (Mahowald 2000). Similarly, subclinical RBD, in which motor tone is disinhibited, has been shown with both acute and chronic administration of serotonergic antidepressants (Winkelman and James 2004).

The diagnosis of RBD is made by polysomnography, which demonstrates elevated muscle tone or excessive phasic muscle activity in the submental and anterior tibialis electromyogram during REM sleep (American Academy of Sleep Medicine, in press). At times, subtle or even gross body movements may be manifest during sleep study. Excess PLMS may also be observed during both REM and non-REM sleep. Otherwise, polysomnographic results are generally normal.

First-line treatment of RBD consists of benzodiazepine receptor agonists (see Table 6–2). The most commonly used agent is clonazepam (0.5–2.0 mg), which has been shown to substantially decrease the number and extent of pathological dream-enacting behaviors (Schenck and Mahowald 1996b). In general, the medication is well tolerated for this indication, although given the older age of most of the patients and the long half-life of this agent, excess daytime sleepiness and/or cognitive impairments may be seen. If these effects occur, shorter-acting benzodiazepines (e.g., lorazepam 1–2 mg) may be utilized. Other medications have also been used with some success, in particular melatonin (3–15 mg qhs) (Boeve et al. 2003a) and pramipexole (0.5–1.0 mg qhs) (Fantini et al. 2003). These alternatives are most attractive in patients for whom a benzodiazepine may be associated with cognitive or motor side effects or those who have a history of substance abuse. Certainly, discontinuation of medications such as serotonergic, tricyclic, or MAOI antidepressants should be attempted when clinically possible. In addition, as with non-REM parasomnias, safety of the sleeping environment for both the patient and the bedpartner is essential.

Nightmare Disorder

Nightmare disorder is characterized by recurrent dreams, usually arising from REM sleep, followed by an awakening from sleep with full recall of the dream. The dominant emotion is usually fear, although anger, sadness, and embarrassment may also be present. Nightmares may occur at any time of night but are more common in the final third of the night, when REM is most prominent (American Academy of Sleep Medicine, in press; Pagel 2000). In distinction to sleep terrors, return to sleep after a nightmare is usually delayed, and frequent nightmares may lead to a fear of going to sleep. Nightmares are not usually associated with acting out of dreams in overt motor behaviors, as occurs in RBD.

Occasional nightmares are common in both children and adults (Nielsen et al. 2000). However, roughly 5% of adults report a history of frequent nightmares (Ohayon et al. 1997; Zadra and Donderi 2000). The prevalence is higher in women than in men, and it is higher in those with a history of a psychiatric disorder. When nightmare distress is assessed independently of nightmare frequency, associations of the former with psychiatric illness and psychopathology are clear (Levin and Fireman 2002). Polysomnography is generally of little diagnostic value for frequent nightmares, although it can rule out RBD and possibly non-REM parasomnias.

Nightmares are present in more than 50% of individuals with posttraumatic stress disorder (PTSD), and in fact are a diagnostic feature of this disorder (Neylan et al. 1998). In individuals with PTSD, the nightmare often has a thematic or literal association with the traumatic event, and recurrent nightmares are not uncommon (Harvey et al. 2003). Nightmares in PTSD are rarely observed in the sleep laboratory, but when observed, they have been seen originating from both REM and non-REM sleep.

A variety of approaches have demonstrated value in the treatment of both trauma-related and non-trauma-related nightmares (Table 6–2). Prazosin (4–12 mg qhs) was effective in one placebo-controlled study (Raskind et al. 2003). In addition, cyproheptadine (Gupta et al. 1998), anticonvulsants (Berlant and van Kammen 2002), and antipsychotic medications (Labbate and Douglas 2000) have been effective in small uncontrolled case series. Imagery rehearsal, in which new versions (with better outcomes) of nightmares are rehearsed during the day, has demonstrated consistent benefit for both trauma-related and non-trauma-related nightmares (Krakow et al. 2001).

Summary

Parasomnias are undesirable behaviors that arise from sleep but are not under full voluntary control. They are divided into those arising from non-REM sleep and those occurring during REM sleep. The former exist along a continuum of behavioral, affective, and autonomic activation. These non-REM parasomnias can produce behaviors that are disturbing, embarrassing, and even dangerous. When indicated, treatment with benzodiazepines is anecdotally effective, although no controlled studies have been performed. The REM-related parasomnias—REM sleep behavior disorder and nightmare disorder—can be idiopathic or can be related to underlying neurologic disorders (synucleinopathies in RBD) or psychiatric disorders (PTSD in nightmare disorder). Treatment with benzodiazepines is beneficial for RBD. Medication or cognitive therapies can be of value in nightmare disorder.

References

American Sleep Disorders Association: International Classification of Sleep Disorders, 2nd Edition. Rochester, MN, American Sleep Disorders Association (in press)

Berlant J, van Kammen DP: Open-label topiramate as primary or adjunctive therapy in chronic civilian posttraumatic stress disorder: a preliminary report. J Clin Psychiatry 63:15–20, 2002

Birketvedt GS, Florholmen J, Sundsfjord J, et al: Behavioral and neuroendocrine characteristics of the night-eating syndrome. JAMA 282:657–663, 1999

Boeve BF, Silber MH, Ferman TJ: Melatonin for treatment of REM sleep behavior disorder in neurologic disorders: results in 14 patients. Sleep Med 4:281–284, 2003a

Boeve BF, Silber MH, Parisi JE, et al: Synucleinopathy pathology and REM sleep behavior disorder plus dementia or parkinsonism. Neurology 61:40–45, 2003b

Bonkalo A: Impulsive acts and confusional states during incomplete arousal from sleep: criminological and forensic implications. Psychiatr Q 48:400–409, 1974

Broughton RJ: Sleep disorders: disorders of arousal? Enuresis, somnambulism, and nightmares occur in confusional states of arousal, not in "dreaming sleep." Science 159:1070–1078, 1968

Cartwright R: Sleepwalking violence: a sleep disorder, a legal dilemma, and a psychological challenge. Am J Psychiatry 161:1149–1158, 2004

Crisp AH: The sleepwalking/night terrors syndrome in adults. Postgrad Med J 72:599–604, 1996

Eisensehr I, Linke R, Noachtar S, et al: Reduced striatal dopamine transporters in idiopathic rapid eye movement sleep behaviour disorder: comparison with Parkinson's disease and controls. Brain 123:1155–1160, 2000

Espa F, Ondze B, Deglise P, et al: Sleep architecture, slow wave activity, and sleep spindles in adult patients with sleepwalking and sleep terrors. Clin Neurophysiol 111:929–939, 2000

Fantini ML, Gagnon JF, Filipini D, et al: The effects of pramipexole in REM sleep behavior disorder. Neurology 61:1418–1420, 2003

Gagnon JF, Fantini ML, Bedard MA, et al: Association between waking EEG slowing and REM sleep behavior disorder in PD without dementia. Neurology 62:401–406, 2004

Gau SF, Soong WT: Psychiatric comorbidity of adolescents with sleep terrors or sleepwalking: a case-control study. Aust N Z J Psychiatry 33:734–739, 1999

Gaudreau H, Joncas S, Zadra A, et al: Dynamics of slow-wave activity during the NREM sleep of sleepwalkers and control subjects. Sleep 23:755–760 [erratum, 23:858], 2000

Gupta S, Popli A, Bathurst E, Hennig, et al: Efficacy of cyproheptadine for nightmares associated with posttraumatic stress disorder. Compr Psychiatry 39:160–164, 1998

Hartman D, Crisp AH, Sedgwick P, et al: Is there a dissociative process in sleepwalking and night terrors? Postgrad Med J 77:244–249, 2001

Harvey AG, Jones C, Schmidt DA: Sleep and posttraumatic stress disorder: a review. Clin Psychol Rev 23:377–407, 2003

Hendricks JC, Morrison AR, Farnbach GL, et al: A disorder of rapid eye movement sleep in a cat. J Am Vet Med Assoc 178:55–57, 1981

Hublin C, Kaprio J, Partinen M, et al: Prevalence and genetics of sleepwalking: a population-based twin study. Neurology 48:177–181, 1997

Hublin C, Kaprio J, Partinen M, et al: Parasomnias: co-occurrence and genetics. Psychiatr Genet 11:65–70, 2001

Joncas S, Zadra A, Paquet J, et al: The value of sleep deprivation as a diagnostic tool in adult sleepwalkers. Neurology 58:936–940, 2002

Kales A, Soldatos CR, Bixler EO, et al: Hereditary factors in sleepwalking and night terrors. Br J Psychiatry 137:111–118, 1980

Kavey NB, Whyte J, Resor SR Jr, et al: Somnambulism in adults. Neurology 40:749–752, 1990

Klump KL, Kaye WH, Strober M: The evolving genetic foundations of eating disorders. Psychiatr Clin North Am 24:215–225, 2001

Krakow B, Hollifield M, Johnston L, et al: Imagery rehearsal therapy for chronic nightmares in sexual assault survivors with posttraumatic stress disorder: a randomized controlled trial. JAMA 286:537–545, 2001

Labbate LA, Douglas S: Olanzapine for nightmares and sleep disturbance in posttraumatic stress disorder (PTSD). Can J Psychiatry 45:667–668, 2000

Laberge L, Tremblay RE, Vitaro F, et al: Development of parasomnias from childhood to early adolescence. Pediatrics 106:67–74, 2000

Landry P, Warnes H, Nielsen T, et al: Somnambulistic-like behaviour in patients attending a lithium clinic. Int Clin Psychopharmacol 14:173–175, 1999

Levin R, Fireman G: Nightmare prevalence, nightmare distress, and self-reported psychological disturbance. Sleep 25:205–212, 2002

Llorente MD, Currier MB, Norman SE, et al: Night terrors in adults: phenomenology and relationship to psychopathology. J Clin Psychiatry 53:392–394, 1992

Mahowald M[W]: Parasomnias, in Principles and Practice of Sleep Medicine, 3rd Edition. Edited by Kryger MH, Roth T, Dement WC. Philadelphia,WB Saunders, 2000, pp 693–796

Mahowald MW: Parasomnias. Med Clin North Am 88:669–678, 2004

Mahowald MW, Schenck CH: Evolving concepts of human state dissociation. Arch Ital Biol 139:269–300, 2001

Marshall HM, Allison KC, O'Reardon JP, et al: Night eating syndrome among nonobese persons. Int J Eat Disord 35:217–222, 2004

Mehlenbeck R, Spirito A, Owens J, et al: The clinical presentation of childhood partial arousal parasomnias. Sleep Med 1:307–312, 2000

Morgenthaler TI, Silber MH: Amnestic sleep-related eating disorder associated with zolpidem. Sleep Med 3:323–327, 2002

Neylan TC, Marmar CR, Metzler TJ, et al: Sleep disturbances in the Vietnam generation: findings from a nationally representative sample of male Vietnam veterans. Am J Psychiatry 155:929–933, 1998

Nielsen TA, Laberge L, Paquet J, et al: Development of disturbing dreams during adolescence and their relation to anxiety symptoms. Sleep 23:727–736, 2000

Ohayon MM, Morselli PL, Guilleminault C: Prevalence of nightmares and their relationship to psychopathology and daytime functioning in insomnia subjects. Sleep 20:340–348, 1997

Ohayon MM, Guilleminault C, Priest RG: Night terrors, sleepwalking, and confusional arousals in the general population: their frequency and relationship to other sleep and mental disorders. J Clin Psychiatry 60:268–276, 1999

Pagel JF: Nightmares and disorders of dreaming. Am Fam Physician 61:2037–2042, 2044, 2000

Raskind MA, Peskind ER, Kanter ED, et al: Reduction of nightmares and other PTSD symptoms in combat veterans by prazosin: a placebo-controlled study. Am J Psychiatry 160:371–373, 2003

Roth B, Nevsimalova S, Rechtschaffen A: Hypersomnia with "sleep drunkenness." Arch Gen Psychiatry 26:456–462, 1972

Schenck CH, Mahowald MW: Long-term, nightly benzodiazepine treatment of injurious parasomnias and other disorders of disrupted nocturnal sleep in 170 adults. Am J Med 100:333–337, 1996a

Schenck CH, Mahowald MW: REM sleep parasomnias. Neurol Clin 14:697–720, 1996b

Schenck CH, Mahowald MW: On the reported association of psychopathology with sleep terrors in adults. Sleep 23:448–449, 2000a

Schenck CH, Mahowald MW: Parasomnias: managing bizarre sleep-related behavior disorders. Postgrad Med 107:145–156, 2000b

Schenck CH, Mahowald MW: REM sleep behavior disorder: clinical, developmental, and neuroscience perspectives 16 years after its formal identification in SLEEP. Sleep 25:120–138, 2002

Schenck CH, Hurwitz TD, Bundlie SR, et al: Sleep-related eating disorders: polysomnographic correlates of a heterogeneous syndrome distinct from daytime eating disorders. Sleep 14:419–431, 1991

Schenck CH, Hurwitz TD, O'Connor KA, et al: Additional categories of sleep-related eating disorders and the current status of treatment. Sleep 16:457–466, 1993

Schenck CH, Bundlie SR, Mahowald MW: Delayed emergence of a parkinsonian disorder in 38% of 29 older men initially diagnosed with idiopathic rapid eye movement sleep behaviour disorder. Neurology 46:388–393 [erratum, 46:1787], 1996

Schenck CH, Boyd JL, Mahowald MW: A parasomnia overlap disorder involving sleepwalking, sleep terrors, and REM sleep behavior disorder in 33 polysomnographically confirmed cases. Sleep 20:972–981, 1997

Shapiro CM, Trajanovic NN, Fedoroff JP: Sexsomnia—a new parasomnia? Can J Psychiatry 48:311–317, 2003

Turner RS, D'Amato CJ, Chervin RD, et al: The pathology of REM sleep behavior disorder with comorbid Lewy body dementia. Neurology 55:1730–1732, 2000

Winkelman JW: Clinical and polysomnographic features of sleep-related eating disorder. J Clin Psychiatry 59:14–19, 1998

Winkelman JW: Treatment of nocturnal eating syndrome and sleep-related eating disorder with topiramate. Sleep Med 4:243–246, 2003

Winkelman JW, James L: Serotonergic antidepressants are associated with REM sleep without atonia. Sleep 27:317–321, 2004

Winkelman JW, Herzog DB, Fava M: The prevalence of sleep-related eating disorder in psychiatric and non-psychiatric populations. Psychol Med 29:1461–1466, 1999

Zadra A, Donderi DC: Nightmares and bad dreams: their prevalence and relationship to well-being. J Abnorm Psychol 109:273–281, 2000

Chapter 7

Circadian Rhythm Sleep Disorders

Phyllis Zee, M.D., Ph.D.
Prasanth Manthena, M.D.

All living organisms on our planet exhibit near 24-hour (circadian) rhythms in physiology and behavior. The sleep-wake cycle is the most striking circadian rhythm in humans. Therefore, it is not surprising that alterations in circadian rhythms are often accompanied by symptoms of insomnia or excessive sleepiness. Recent advances in our understanding of basic human circadian biology have led to the development of new approaches for the diagnosis and treatment of circadian rhythm sleep disorders (CRSDs). Therefore, in this chapter we will provide a brief review of the current knowledge of the neurobiology of circadian rhythms and how the circadian system responds to photic as well as to nonphotic entraining agents.

In mammals, these self-sustaining circadian rhythms are generated by a master pacemaker, the suprachiasmatic nucleus (SCN), a paired structure located in the hypothalamus (Moore and Eichler 1972; Stephan and Zucker 1972). In the 1990s, one of the most important advances in biology was the elucidation of the molecular basis of circadian timing. Through feedback loops at the transcription and translation levels, circadian clock proteins oscillate, generating a self-sustaining timing system (Dunlap 1999). This timing system, in turn, is responsible for the organism's endogenous circadian rhythm. When all external time cues are taken away (e.g., placing a human in a dark cave without access to the outside world), this endogenous rhythm can be observed by following the sleep-wake cycle and markers such as dim-light melatonin onset (DLMO) and core body temperature, which follow a strong circadian pattern.

The circadian free-running period (length of the cycle of endogenous rhythm oscillation) has been shown to be largely genetically determined, with some interspecies and individual differences. In both the mouse and the hamster, genes have been identified that lengthen and shorten the free-running period (Ralph and Menaker 1988; Vitaterna et al. 1994; Zheng et al. 1999). The mammalian circadian period is generally slightly longer than 24 hours in diurnal animals and slightly shorter than 24 hours in nocturnal animals. In humans, the average circadian period has been estimated to be approximately 24.2 hours and to require daily alignment with the 24-hour external environment (Czeisler et al. 1999).

The SCN not only generates circadian rhythms, but also synchronizes the free-running rhythm to the external physical environment (Moore 1997). The process of synchronizing the endogenous rhythm of an individual to the 24-hour day is referred to as *entrainment.* Light, physical activity, and social activity can entrain circadian rhythms (Figure 7–1). In humans, light is the strongest synchronizing agent for the circadian clock (Czeisler et al. 1986). The direction and magnitude of the effects of light are strongly dependent on the timing of exposure. Light in the first half of the night delays circadian rhythms, whereas light late in the second half of the night or in the early morning advances circadian rhythms. In humans, the transition point between the delay and advance regions occurs near the temperature minimum (4:00 A.M. to 6:00 A.M.) in young adults and somewhat earlier in older adults (Boivin et al. 1994; Minors et al. 1991). The magnitude of the phase shift caused by light at any given time point can be graphically represented as a phase response curve (Figure 7–2). Recent evidence indicates that the primary circadian photoreceptors are melanopsin-containing retinal ganglion cells. These distinct cells play little to no role in visual perception and project through the retinohypothalamic tract, instead of the optic tracts, to reach the hypothalamus (Bellingham and Foster 2002; Miyamoto and Sancar 1998).

Although full-spectrum bright light is a strong and reliable entraining agent of circadian rhythms, recent evidence indicates

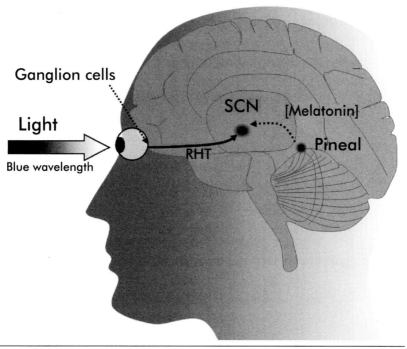

Figure 7–1. Components of the human circadian timing system.
The suprachiasmatic nucleus (SCN) is the dominant "clock" in humans. It can be synchronized (entrained) to the outside world by several means. The most powerful entraining agent is light (particularly light in the blue spectrum). Melanopsin-containing ganglion cells in the retina (distinct from the rods and cones) are the main circadian photoreceptors and project through the retinohypothalamic tract to the SCN. The SCN also receives a smaller input from the retina through the lateral geniculate body (not shown). The SCN can also be modulated by agents such as melatonin, which is secreted with a strong circadian rhythm from the pineal gland.

that lower intensities, such as those encountered in ordinary room lighting, can also affect the timing of human circadian rhythms (Zeitzer et al. 2000). The recent discovery that both light-induced phase shifts and melatonin suppression are most sensitive to short-wavelength light of approximately 460 nm provides an exciting new avenue for the development of light therapies to treat circadian rhythm sleep disorders (Lockley et al. 2003; Warman et al. 2003). With the use of blue light emitters (i.e., short-wavelength light), phase shifting of circadian rhythms may be possible with briefer and less intense light exposure.

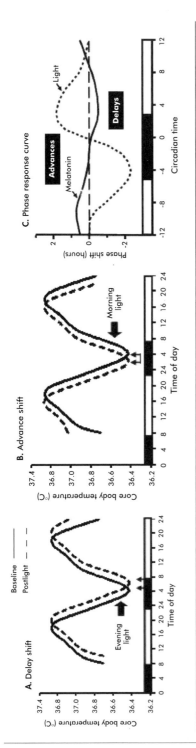

Figure 7–2. Phase response curve.

A and B: Several physiological processes can be used as circadian rhythm markers. In panels A and B, core body temperature is graphed with respect to time of day. Temperature is often used in circadian rhythm research because of its marked circadian rhythm (peaking during the day and reaching its nadir in the morning). Here the effects of evening light delaying the temperature rhythm and morning light advancing the temperature rhythm are shown. The magnitude of phase shift caused by light can then be plotted to create a phase response curve. **C:** Plotting the magnitude of phase shift caused by light at any given time point creates a phase response curve. At time point 0 (typically the temperature minimum in most young subjects), light has no effect on circadian rhythm. Before this time point, light delays the circadian rhythm; after it, light advances the circadian rhythm. Note how the presence of light at certain time points can cause a dramatic shift in the phase of the circadian rhythm, whereas at other time points (midday) it has little to no effect. Also, note that the effects of other synchronizing agents, such as melatonin, can also be plotted as a phase response curve.

The role of nonphotic cues as synchronizing agents for the human circadian system has been recognized since the early 1970s when Aschoff and colleagues (1971) demonstrated that scheduled bedtimes, mealtimes, and other social cues could entrain circadian rhythms. More recent studies have shown that physical exercise during the night can produce a phase delay in human circadian rhythms (Baehr et al. 2003; Buxton et al. 1997). These findings suggest that timed structured social and physical activities may have a role in the management of circadian rhythm sleep disorders.

There is substantial evidence that melatonin, secreted with a strong circadian rhythm by the pineal gland, is another important modulator of circadian rhythms and sleep. Administration of exogenous melatonin to humans in the early evening advances the phase of the circadian rhythms, whereas administration in the early morning delays the phase. The greatest and most consistent phase-shifting effects of melatonin occur during the evening, just preceding the increase in endogenous melatonin levels (Cajochen et al. 2003; Lewy et al. 1998). In addition to its phase-resetting properties, melatonin appears to modulate sleep and wakefulness by increasing evening sleep propensity and reducing core body temperature (Cajochen et al. 2003) (see Figure 7–1 and Figure 7–2). On the basis of its phase-shifting and sleep-modulating effects, melatonin has been proposed for the treatment of several circadian rhythm sleep disorders, including the delayed sleep phase type and the nonentrained type.

Our current understanding of the regulation of the human sleep and wake cycle indicates that sleep and wake states are generated by a complex interaction of endogenous circadian (C) and sleep homeostatic (S) processes. This two-process interaction is modified by social and environmental factors. Process S can be conceptualized as an hourglass mechanism relating the amount and intensity of sleep to the duration of prior wakefulness. Therefore, process S accumulates (increasing drive for sleep) as a function of wake time and decreases with sleep. The circadian clock (process C) plays an essential role in the maintenance of wakefulness during the day and thus also in consolidation of sleep during the night (Czeisler et al. 1980; Dijk and Czeisler

1994; Zulley et al. 1981). It is likely that the SCN exerts its alerting effects via output pathways to areas in the hypothalamus that play a role in increasing arousal, such as the dorsomedial and posterior hypothalamus (Berk and Finkelstein 1981). In most individuals, there is a midday dip in alertness occurring at around 2:00 to 4:00 in the afternoon, followed by an increase in alertness that gradually reaches a peak during the early to midevening hours, and then a decline to its lowest levels between 4:00 and 6:00 in the morning. Despite the homeostatic drive for sleep being the highest in the evening, maximum alertness occurs at this time because the circadian signal for alertness is also at its peak during these hours (Figure 7–3) (Carskadon and Dement 1975, 1977; Dantz et al. 1994; Dijk and Czeisler 1995; Strogatz et al. 1987). The normal interaction between the homeostatic and circadian processes results in a wake period of approximately 16 hours and a sleep period of 8 hours.

Alterations in the regulation of the circadian timing system or a misalignment between the endogenous circadian rhythm and the external physical or social environment can affect the timing or duration of sleep and give rise to circadian rhythm sleep disorders. In this chapter, the classification and diagnostic criteria for CRSD and its subtypes are based on the revised *International Classification of Sleep Disorders,* 2nd Edition (ICSD-2) (American Academy of Sleep Medicine, in press) and DSM-IV-TR (American Psychiatric Association 2000). Table 7–1 summarizes the primary CRSDs.

Delayed Sleep Phase Type

(In DSM-IV-TR, the pertinent classification is *circadian rhythm sleep disorder, delayed sleep phase type.* In ICSD-2, it is *delayed sleep phase type.*)

Delayed sleep phase type (DSPT) was the first CRSD to be described and is also the most common (Yamadera et al. 1996). DSPT patients typically have difficulty falling asleep before 2:00 A.M. to 6:00 A.M. and have difficulty waking up before 10:00 A.M. to 1:00 P.M. (Weitzman et al. 1981). When DSPT patients are allowed to sleep at their preferred sleep-wake times, they have normal sleep

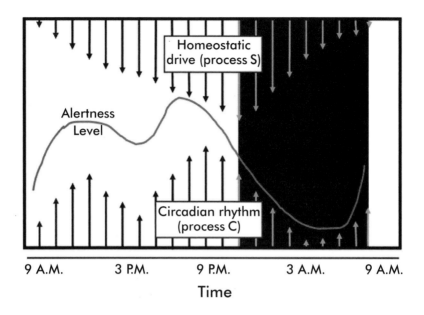

Figure 7–3. The two-process model.
Alertness level is determined by the interaction between two processes. The sleep homeostatic drive (process S) promotes sleep and builds up during wake, reaching a maximum in the late evening (near the usual sleep time). The circadian rhythm system (process C) promotes wakefulness during the day. It is biphasic and tends to dip in the midafternoon. Process C also reaches its peak in the evening, to counterbalance the accumulation of homeostatic drive that has built up throughout the day, and it begins to fall just before the usual bedtime. This system promotes wakefulness during the day and consolidates sleep at night. Dark area represents sleep time.

architecture and quality. But when attempting to keep aligned with societal norms, these patients tend to have sleep-onset insomnia and excessive daytime sleepiness (EDS), especially during the morning hours (Regestein and Monk 1995). The preferences of DSPT patients to have delayed sleep-wake times remain stable over a long period of time, unlike the short-lived preferences seen, for example, after jet lag or shift work. On measures such as the Horne-Ostberg questionnaire (Horne and Ostberg 1976), both DSPT patients and evening types ("owls") show preferences for being more alert during the late evening hours. However, in addition to being evening types, DSPT patients are less able to adjust their sleep-wake times, resulting in complaints of insomnia or ex-

Table 7–1. The primary circadian rhythm sleep disorders

Type	Typical sleep-wake times[a]	Patient population	Treatment options
Delayed sleep phase type	Delayed bed/wake times Bedtime: 2:00–6:00 A.M. Wake time: 10:00 A.M.–1:00 P.M.	More commonly found in adolescents	*Melatonin:* 5–10 mg, 5 h before bedtime *Bright light therapy:* Morning: 1–2 h, 2,000–10,000 lux *Chronotherapy:* Progressively delay bedtimes
Advanced sleep phase type	Advanced bed/wake times Bedtime: 6:00–9:00 P.M. Wake time: 2:00–5:00 A.M.	Rare; especially unusual in the young; more common in older adults	*Bright light therapy:* Evening: 1–2 h, 2,000–10,000 lux *Chronotherapy:* Progressively advance bedtimes
Nonentrained type	Bedtimes and wake times progressively occur at a later time each day	High prevalence in the blind; very rare in sighted individuals	*Melatonin:* 10 mg before desired bedtime *Structured activity:* Maintain a regular schedule
Irregular sleep-wake type	No regular bedtimes or wake times: frequent short naps throughout the day and night	Most commonly seen in patients with underlying neurologic dysfunction, e.g., head trauma, dementia	*Bright light:* Morning bright light *Structured activity:* Increase physical and social activity during the day

[a]When patients are allowed to sleep at their desired times without social restrictions.

cessive sleepiness (Dagan 2002; Horne and Ostberg 1976).

Of particular relevance to psychiatry is the high prevalence of affective disorders (Schrader et al. 1996) and personality disorders in patients with DSPT. Furthermore, there is some evidence to suggest that DSPT is also more common in patients with personality disorders (Dagan et al. 1996, 1998). In addition, the psychological profile and personality features of DSPT patients are similar to those found in neurosis and depression (Shirayama et al. 2003). Both affective disorders and these personality features of DSPT can contribute to social withdrawal. It has been proposed that social withdrawal can lead to a decrease in light exposure, physical activity, and social cues. This reduced exposure to circadian rhythm entraining cues may thus perpetuate DSPT.

Epidemiology

The prevalence of DSPT in the general population has been estimated to be less than 1% (Wagner 1996). However, DSPT is more common among adolescents, with a reported prevalence of 7%–16% (Pelayo et al. 1988). It is estimated that approximately 7% of patients with chronic insomnia presenting to a sleep clinic have DSPT (Weitzman et al. 1981).

Pathophysiology and Etiology

Although the exact pathophysiology of DSPT is unknown, a disruption of the circadian timing system or an alteration in the interaction between the circadian and homeostatic sleep- and wake-regulating processes has been postulated to play an essential role. There is also growing evidence of a genetic basis for DSPT. For example, a positive family history is not uncommon, and one large family with DSPT has been reported (Ancoli-Israel et al. 2001). Furthermore, polymorphisms in circadian genes such as *PER3*, arylalkylamine *N*-acetyltransferase (*AANAT*), *HLA*, and *CLOCK* have been shown to be associated with DSPT (Archer et al. 2003; Ebisawa et al. 2001; Hohjoh et al. 2003; Iwase et al. 2002; Takahashi et al. 2000).

Several mechanisms based on the principles of circadian biology could account for a persistently delayed sleep phase. One possibility is that patients with DSPT have an unusually long endogenous circadian period (Regestein and Monk 1995). It is possible that the greater frequency of longer circadian periods in adolescents (Carskadon et al. 1999) may be related to a higher prevalence of DSPT in this population (Regestein and Monk 1995). Another explanation for a persistently delayed phase is an alteration in circadian entrainment by light. For example, individuals with DSPT may have unusually small advance regions (morning) or unusually large delay regions (evening) of the phase response curve to light (Weitzman et al. 1981), resulting in the inability to advance their circadian rhythms. In addition, changes in light sensitivity may play a role in the pathogenesis of DSPT; individuals with DSPT appear to be hypersensitive to nighttime light (Aoki et al. 2001). In addition to alterations in the circadian system, behavioral factors such as evening exposure to light and lack of early-morning light exposure (due to prolonged sleep in the morning) often contribute to the delayed sleep phase under normal light/dark cycles (Ozaki et al. 1996).

Although it is commonly accepted that sleep architecture is essentially normal in patients with DSPT (Alvarez et al. 1992; Thorpy et al. 1988; Uchiyama et al. 1992; Weitzman et al. 1981), there is increasing evidence that changes in the homeostatic regulation of sleep may contribute to the symptoms of insomnia and sleepiness. Uchiyama and colleagues (1999, 2000) have shown that following sleep deprivation, DSPT patients have decreased ability to compensate for sleep loss during the day and the first few hours of the night.

Assessment and Diagnosis

Diagnosis of DSPT is based on a stable delay of the major sleep period (typically until later than 1:00 A.M.) and a history of chronic or recurrent inability to fall asleep and awaken at conventional or socially acceptable times. Patients with DSPT are distinguished from "evening types" or "owls" by the fact that sleep disturbance is associated with impairment of social, occupational, or other areas of function. Although polysomnography is not required for the diagnosis, it may be useful to exclude other sleep disorders.

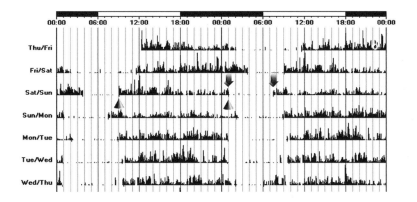

Figure 7–4. A typical rest-activity record from a patient with circadian rhythm disorder, delayed sleep phase type (DSPT), recorded using wrist actigraphy.

This device uses a motion detector, and when the subject is awake (area between the two cones) it records a much greater amount of movement than when the subject is sleeping (area between the two arrows). In this DSPT patient, the bedtime is stably delayed until after 1:00 A.M. throughout the week. Note that on weekends there is a greater delay in the patient's bedtime compared with weekdays.

In addition to the history, diagnostic procedures such as sleep logs, actigraphy, and physiological markers of circadian phase may aid in confirming the diagnosis. Sleep logs or actigraphy monitoring (actigraphy is done by using a wrist-mounted motion detector and sleep logs) for at least 7 days will demonstrate a stable delay in the timing of the habitual sleep and wake times (Figure 7–4). Evaluation of sleep and wake patterns during the weekend or nonworking days usually will reveal sleep and wake times that are later than during weekdays. When the diagnosis is in question, physiological markers of circadian phase, such as dim-light salivary melatonin onset or the nadir of the core body temperature rhythm, are often useful for confirmation of the delayed circadian phase (see Figure 7–2).

Screening for psychiatric disorders and the use of psychoactive medications should be routinely conducted as part of the evaluation for suspected DSPT. For example, the development of DSPT has been associated with the use of fluvoxamine, where either discontinuation of the drug or treatment with melatonin corrected the sleep disorder (Dagan 2002). Also, similar to other populations with chronic symptoms of insomnia and excessive sleepiness, individuals with DSPT may use alcohol, sedative-hypnotics, and stimulants to alleviate symptoms, which may lead to substance dependence.

Treatment

Treatment approaches for DSPT include chronotherapy, timed bright light, and melatonin. Treatment success depends on many variables, including severity of the delayed sleep phase, comorbid psychopathology, ability and willingness of the patient to comply with treatment, school schedule, work obligations, and social pressures (Ohta et al. 1992; Regestein and Monk 1995; Thorpy et al. 1988).

Chronotherapy is a behavioral approach in which the bedtime is delayed (i.e., moved to a later clock time) by approximately 3 hours every 2 days until the desired sleep time is achieved (Weitzman et al. 1981). Most patients will need to be free of social and work requirements for at least 1 week and must adhere to a strict sleep-wake schedule. In addition, light exposure must be carefully controlled. This approach can be effective, but the strict protocol and the length of treatment may limit its acceptability in clinical practice. However, in children, and particularly among adolescents, where behavioral factors likely contribute to the high prevalence of the delayed sleep phase, chronotherapy with its emphasis on adherence to a strict sleep and wake schedule is often useful.

Bright light exposure during the early morning hours is an accepted and effective treatment for DSPT (Chesson et al. 1999). Rosenthal and colleagues (1990) showed that after 2 weeks of exposure to bright light in the morning (2 hours each day at an intensity of 2,500 lux) and avoidance of evening light, individuals with DSPT fell asleep earlier and were more alert in the morning. Although the timing, intensity, and duration of light treatment remain to be defined, exposure to broad-spectrum light of 2,000–10,000 lux for approximately 1–2 hours shortly after awakening in the morning is generally recommended. As with other types of behavioral therapies, compliance with daily or chronic intermittent exposure to light may be problematic. One important factor that affects compliance is the inability of patients to wake up in the morning for light exposure (Thorpy et al. 1988). With the discovery that the blue wavelength of light is in large part responsible for the phase shifts seen after phototherapy, research is currently being done to determine whether blue light emitters can decrease the intensity and duration of bright light therapy. Compliance with bright light therapy will likely increase with shorter duration and lower intensity of light exposure.

Because behavioral and bright light therapies have limitations, pharmacologic approaches for the treatment of DSPT have been increasingly studied. Melatonin, a hormone produced by the pineal gland, has circadian phase-shifting effects and also acts as a mild hypnotic. Several small clinical trials have shown that melatonin (typically 5 mg) administered in the evening can advance both sleep onset and wake times and improve quality of life of DSPT patients (Dahlitz et al. 1991; Nagtegaal et al. 2000; Oldani et al. 1994). However, because of the variable timing of administration and dose between studies and the relative lack of large-scale controlled clinical trials, clinical guidelines for the use of melatonin are not available. Although melatonin is widely used as an over-the-counter nutritional supplement to improve sleep, patients should be advised regarding potential adverse effects. Melatonin has been shown to have vasoactive properties (peripheral vasodilation, cerebrovascular vasoconstriction) and may have antigonadal effects. Thus, caution needs to taken when considering melatonin for use in children and pregnant women (Burgess et al. 2002).

Other pharmacologic agents have also been tried in the treatment of DSPT. In a small number of trials and case reports, hypnotics have been shown to advance sleep time. However, in some patients they did not advance wake times, and in a few cases hypnotic use appeared to worsen depressive symptoms (Ozaki et al. 1989; Regestein and Pavlova 1995). Literature is also scarce regarding the use of stimulants. Methylphenidate, in a small case series, has been reported to relieve symptoms of excessive daytime sleepiness when given 1 hour before desired wake time (Salin-

Pascual et al. 1988). Clearly, more studies are needed to clarify the role, if any, of hypnotics and stimulants in the treatment of DSPT.

Advanced Sleep Phase Type

(In DSM-IV-TR, the pertinent classification is *circadian rhythm sleep disorder, unspecified type, advanced sleep phase pattern*. In ICSD-2, it is *advanced sleep phase type*.)

Advanced sleep phase type (ASPT) is characterized by habitual sleep-wake times that are several hours earlier relative to desired and conventional times (Figure 7–5). Compared with DSPT patients who cannot fall asleep until after their desired bedtimes, ASPT patients fall asleep earlier than desired. Individuals with ASPT typically report sleep onset of 6:00–9:00 P.M. and wake time of 2:00–5:00 A.M. (Kamei et al. 1998; Moldofsky et al. 1986). When they attempt to maintain a conventional schedule, their most common complaints are early morning awakenings, sleep maintenance insomnia (once asleep, the inability to stay asleep), and excessive sleepiness in the late afternoon or early evening. However, when these individuals are allowed to follow an advanced schedule, sleep architecture and quality are usually normal for age. Use of alcohol, sedative-hypnotics, or stimulants to treat symptoms of sleep-maintenance insomnia and daytime sleepiness may lead to substance abuse.

Epidemiology

The actual prevalence of ASPT in the general population is unknown, but it has been estimated to be about 1% in middle-aged and older adults (Ando et al. 1995). The circadian rhythm tends to advance with age. There are only a few case reports of patients with ASPT that are not associated with this aging process (Jones et al. 1999; Moldofsky et al. 1986; Reid et al. 2001). One possible explanation for this may be that it is more socially acceptable to be an "early bird" who arrives at work ahead of time rather than a "night owl" who may chronically arrive late. Therefore, patients with an advanced sleep phase may not consider their sleep habits an impairment that requires medical attention.

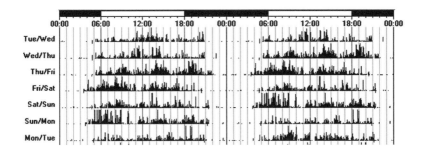

Figure 7–5. A typical rest-activity record from a patient with circadian rhythm disorder, advanced sleep phase type, recorded using wrist actigraphy.

The bedtime is advanced to about 8:00 P.M. and wake time to about 5:00–6:00 A.M. in this patient.

Pathophysiology and Etiology

Although the precise mechanisms underlying the pathophysiology of ASPT, like those of DSPT, are not completely understood, evidence strongly indicates an alteration in the circadian timing system itself or in the interaction between the circadian system and sleep homeostatic regulation. Circadian-based mechanisms, such as an unusually short endogenous circadian period or alterations in the entrainment process of the circadian system, may result in an advanced sleep phase (Ancoli-Israel and Kripke 1991; Jones et al. 1999; Moore 1999; Naylor et al. 2000). There is also evidence that the interaction between circadian timing and sleep homeostatic regulation may be altered in older adults with advanced sleep phase (Duffy and Czeisler 2002).

Genetic factors have been found to play an important role in the pathogenesis of ASPT. Several families with ASPT have been identified (Jones et al. 1999; Reid et al. 2001; Satoh et al. 2003). A mutation in the *PER2* gene that results in decreased phosphorylation of the PER2 protein was identified in one family (Toh et al. 2001). This mutation was associated with a shortened circadian rhythm period in one of the affected members (Jones et al. 1999). However, this *PER2* mutation was not found in other families with ASPT, indicating genetic heterogeneity of the condition (Satoh et al. 2003).

Assessment and Diagnosis

A clinical history of chronic or recurrent early evening sleepiness and early morning awakening that is associated with an advance in the timing of the major sleep period (relative to desired or conventional times) is characteristic of ASPT. In addition to the history, a sleep log diary or actigraphy over a period of at least 7 days can be used to confirm the diagnosis by demonstrating a stable advance in the timing of the habitual sleep period. Circadian rhythm markers such as melatonin and core body temperature are often measured to document an advanced phase in research settings, but these measures are not readily available in clinical practice. Other psychiatric or sleep disorders that may produce alterations in the sleep-wake cycle should be excluded. Therefore, a careful history to exclude affective disorders such as depression, primary insomnia, and sleep-disordered breathing is necessary. Because a common complaint among depressed patients is early morning awakening, it is important to distinguish ASPT from major depression and other affective disorders (Wagner 1996). Although polysomnography is not required for the diagnosis, it may be useful as a way to identify other sleep disorders.

Treatment

Treatment approaches for ASPT, as for DSPT, may include chronotherapy, exposure to light in the evening, and pharmacotherapy. Chronotherapy for ASPT requires progressively advancing the sleep time (i.e., moving it to an earlier clock time) by 2 hours every 2 days until the desired sleep time is achieved (Moldofsky et al. 1986). As mentioned earlier, because of the behavioral restrictions, the use of chronotherapy has been limited in clinical practice.

Bright light is the most commonly used treatment for ASPT. Exposure to evening bright light (7:00–9:00 P.M.) has been shown to successfully delay circadian rhythms (Lack and Schumacher 1993). Bright light exposure in the evening improved sleep efficiency and delayed the phase of circadian rhythms, but patients had difficulty maintaining the treatment regimen (Campbell

1999). Exposure to evening light should be accompanied by avoidance of bright light in the early morning hours, because light exposure at this time serves to further advance circadian rhythms (Crowley et al. 2003). Theoretically, melatonin if given in the morning could also delay circadian rhythms and could be used to treat ASPT. However, there is a lack of empirical data documenting its usefulness in the treatment of ASPT. Furthermore, potential residual sedative effects of melatonin administered in the morning could be a limiting factor. Other agents, such as hypnotics and stimulants, have not been systematically studied.

Nonentrained Type

(In DSM-IV-TR, the pertinent category is *circadian rhythm sleep disorder, unspecified type, non-24-hour sleep-wake pattern, free-running type*. In ICSD-2, it is *non-24-hour sleep-wake type*.)

Nonentrained type is typically characterized by a daily delay of the major sleep period that corresponds to the endogenous period of the circadian clock. In these individuals, the circadian clock is not entrained or is weakly entrained to the physical and social 24-hour cycle (Figure 7–6), so that sleep starts progressively later each day. When the circadian timing for sleep and wakefulness is aligned to the external physical and social environment, sleep quality and duration are typically normal. However, because the endogenous period of the human circadian clock is slightly longer than 24 hours (Czeisler et al. 1999), the timing of sleep will delay and eventually will become out of phase with the desired or conventional times. Because of the continuous drift, when attempts are made to keep conventional sleep-wake times, these patients present with complaints of insomnia or excessive sleepiness that may vary from week to week.

Epidemiology

Nonentrained type CRSD was originally described in blind people, with an estimated prevalence of 50% (Miles et al. 1977; Sack et al. 1992). There have been only a few reports of the nonentrained type in sighted individuals (McArthur et al. 1996).

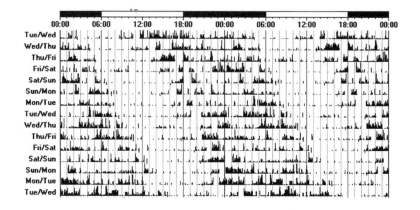

Figure 7–6. A typical rest-activity record from a patient with circadian rhythm disorder, nonentrained type, recorded using wrist actigraphy. The major sleep period is not entrained to the 24-hour day and chronically drifts, with a further short delay each day.

Pathophysiology and Etiology

The high prevalence of nonentrained circadian rhythms in blind people is most likely due to the lack of photic entrainment. However, in blind people who have entrained circadian rhythms, scheduled social or physical activities may serve as synchronizing agents to maintain entrainment. Interestingly, there is evidence that the circadian system in some blind individuals (without visual light perception) can still respond to bright light (Czeisler et al. 1995). This finding is consistent with the more recent evidence that the receptors predominantly responsible for the circadian photic responses are different from those for vision. The retinal ganglion cells, rather than the rods and cones, are predominantly responsible for the circadian phase–shifting effects of light. Also, the retinohypothalamic tract, which contains the projections from these photoreceptors, is distinct from the optic pathways responsible for vision (Guido et al. 2002; Lockley et al. 2003; Menaker 2003; Warman et al. 2003).

In sighted individuals, the etiology is less clear. One possible explanation is that these individuals may have an extremely prolonged endogenous circadian period that is outside the range of entrainment to the 24-hour day (Uchiyama et al. 2002). Supporting this hypothesis are reports of DSPT patients (presumably with long intrinsic circadian period) who developed a nonentrained sleep-wake pattern during phase-delay chronotherapy (Oren and Wehr 1992). As with DSPT, alterations in the response of the circadian system to synchronizing agents such as light could result in weakened entrainment or lack of entrainment of the circadian rhythms (McArthur et al. 1996). Delayed sleep propensity relative to the phase of the circadian clock in sighted individuals with nonentrained circadian rhythms, as reported by Uchiyama and colleagues (2002) could potentially result in accelerated light-induced phase delays.

Assessment and Diagnosis

The diagnosis of a nonentrained CRSD requires a history of periodic complaints of insomnia or excessive sleepiness associated with the lack of a stable entrainment of the circadian sleep-wake cycle to the 24-hour physical environment. In addition, actigraphy and sleep logs are useful diagnostic tools in the evaluation and often will help confirm the nonentrained pattern. Actigraphy and sleep logs should be recorded for at least 2 weeks so that the typical progressive daily delay drift in the timing of sleep and wake can be seen. When actigraphy is not available, sleep logs, along with a history of daytime napping and periodic insomnia, can accurately predict nonentrained CRSD in blind people (Sack and Lewy 2001). Although polysomnography is not required for the diagnosis, it may be useful in evaluating for other sleep disorders. Results will vary depending on the time of the sleep recording. If sleep data for a patient with nonentrained type are recorded at a time when the patient's circadian sleep propensity coincides with the conventional clock hours, the results should be essentially normal for age.

In sighted people, social and behavioral factors, such as irregular schedules and medical, neurologic, and psychiatric disorders should be considered. There is an increased incidence of psychiatric and personality disorders in patients with nonentrained type (McArthur et al. 1996). Particularly in patients with cognitive impairments, lack of exposure to regular social schedules and light/dark schedules may result in what appears to be a nonentrained sleep-wake cycle (Palm et al. 1997).

Treatment

Several approaches using behavioral strategies, such as timed, regular schedules of sleep and social and work activities that are aimed to entrain circadian rhythms, have been shown to be useful in the management of this condition in blind people. When structured activity is insufficient to maintain entrainment, melatonin has been shown to be effective. A melatonin dose of 10 mg, typically taken 1 hour before bedtime, has been shown to entrain the timing of sleep in blind people (Sack et al. 2000). After a gradual titration down from a starting dose of 10 mg, as little as 0.5 mg of melatonin was sufficient to maintain entrainment (Lewy et al. 2001).

Much less information is available regarding the management of sighted individuals with nonentrained type. Strategies to increase the strength of both photic and nonphotic synchronizing agents may be useful (McArthur et al. 1996). It has been suggested that flurazepam and vitamin B_{12} may be effective in some individuals (Kamgar-Parsi et al. 1983). The available data in blind people suggest that melatonin in the evening and/or bright light exposure during the day to reinforce entrainment are reasonable approaches for the management of the condition in sighted persons.

Irregular Sleep-Wake Type

(In DSM-IV-TR, the pertinent classification is *circadian rhythm sleep disorder, unspecified type, irregular sleep-wake pattern*. In ICSD-2, it is *irregular sleep-wake pattern*.)

Irregular sleep-wake type is characterized by lack of a major sleep or wake period during a typical 24-hour day. Patients with this disorder have a complaint of insomnia and/or excessive sleepiness associated with usually three or more irregular naps over a 24-hour period. Normally each nap last a few hours. A near-24-hour sleep-wake rhythm is not discernible in these patients.

Epidemiology

Although originally described in cognitively intact patients who had spent years bedridden and isolated because of prolonged illness, this disorder is most commonly seen in patients with underlying neurologic dysfunction, such as children with psychomotor retardation, traumatic brain injury, and elderly people with dementia (Hoogendijk et al. 1996; Wagner 1996; Witting et al. 1990).

Pathophysiology and Etiology

It is postulated that the underlying pathophysiology is a low amplitude or irregular circadian rhythm due to dysfunction of the central processes responsible for the generation of circadian rhythms. Structural changes in the hypothalamus and the circadian pacemaker (SCN) have been implicated in the etiology of irregular sleep and wake pattern in patients with Alzheimer's disease (Hoogendijk et al. 1996). Populations in which irregular sleep-wake patterns are most common are also those who tend to have decreased exposure to synchronizing agents, such as light and activity (Pollak and Stokes 1997; van Someren et al. 1996). Therefore, both circadian dysfunction and decreased exposure to environmental synchronizing signals most likely are involved in the development and maintenance of irregular or arrhythmic sleep and wake patterns.

Assessment and Diagnosis

Diagnosis is primarily made on the basis of clinical history. However, continuous monitoring of sleep and wake patterns with wrist actigraphy or sleep logs for a minimum of 1 week can confirm an irregular or undetectable circadian rhythm. A careful history should be taken to exclude other sleep disorders and psychiatric disorders in which sleep and wake cycles may be disrupted, such as posttraumatic stress disorder (Dagan 2002). In addition, the history should include information about the patient's daily routine and schedule so that irregular sleep-wake type can be distinguished from poor sleep hygiene and voluntary maintenance of irregular sleep schedules. In elderly individuals with dementia, incontinence and sleep apnea should also be considered.

Treatment

The treatment of irregular sleep-wake type is aimed at consolidating nocturnal sleep. This can be accomplished by strengthening circadian synchronizing agents and by promoting wakefulness during the day. Some methods to consolidate sleep and cycles include increasing exposure to bright light in the morning, minimizing light and noise at night, and structuring social and physical activities (Ancoli-Israel et al. 2002; Naylor et al. 2000; Okawa et al. 1991; Schnelle et al. 1998; Van Someren et al. 1999). A trial using a combination of bright light, chronotherapy, vitamin B_{12}, and hypnotics demonstrated that 45% of patients with irregular sleep cycles responded to this treatment (Yamadera et al. 1996). In children with psychomotor retardation, melatonin given in the evening can improve sleep and wake patterns (Pillar et al. 2000). The role of melatonin in the treatment of this condition has not been established in children or adults. Despite the potential usefulness of both pharmacologic and behavioral strategies, treatment of patients with this disorder needs to be individualized, and success is highly variable.

Shift Work Type

(In DSM-IV-TR, the pertinent category is *circadian rhythm sleep disorder, shift work type*. In ICSD-2, it is *shift work type*.)

Shift work type circadian rhythm disorder is characterized by excessive sleepiness that occurs when work hours are scheduled during the usual sleep period (when the circadian alerting signal is low) and insomnia when attempting to sleep during the usual wake period (when circadian alertness is high). Shift work sleep disorder is most commonly seen in association with night and early morning shift schedules. Patients report decreased total sleep time, poor sleep quality, and impaired performance at work (Akerstedt 1995, 2003; Knauth et al. 1980). Because of decreased alertness, safety at work and during the commute home is a major concern for these individuals.

Epidemiology

In industrialized countries, approximately 20% of the workforce is employed in jobs that require nonstandard work schedules (Presser 1999). Although sleep complaints may be common among shift workers, the actual prevalence of sleep and wakefulness disturbances that are clinically significant and caused by work schedules is unknown (Reinberg et al. 1989). A reasonable estimate, based on data available for night shift workers, is that 5% of the population is affected by this CRSD (Akerstedt 2003).

Pathophysiology and Etiology

The underlying pathophysiology of disturbed sleep and wakefulness due to shift work is misalignment between the time when the worker is required to be awake and the worker's need to sleep as determined by the circadian rhythm of alertness and sleep propensity. Even among permanent night workers, the timing of internal circadian rhythms is usually out of phase with the desired sleep-wake times (Dumont et al. 2001). The excessive sleepiness is likely the result of both decreased circadian alertness during the work period and chronic accumulated sleep loss.

Assessment and Diagnosis

Shift work type circadian rhythm disorder can be usually diagnosed by a history of insomnia and excessive sleepiness that occur in relation to shift work and persist for the duration of the shift work. Typically the sleep disturbance improves when the individual resumes a more conventional work schedule, but in some individuals, the sleep disturbance may persist. Diagnostic tests such as sleep logs and actigraphy are useful in demonstrating disturbed sleep and napping behavior. If the history suggests common comorbid disorders, such as sleep apnea, a polysomnogram to evaluate this possibility is recommended. When objective evaluation of the level of sleepiness is indicated, such as in situations in which safety is of significant concern, the multiple sleep latency test or maintenance of wakefulness test can be used during work hours (Littner et al. 2005).

In addition to sleep disturbances, shift work has been associated with increased prevalence of both medical and psychiatric disorders (Wagner 1996). Increased association with cardiovascular and gastrointestinal disorders, sleep apnea, obesity, and miscarriage has been reported in shift workers (Scott 2000). Use of sedatives, stimulants, and alcohol should be considered as contributing factors because many shift workers self-medicate to alleviate symptoms (Wagner 1996). In terms of psychiatric illnesses, mood disorders have been specifically linked with shift work. Studies have shown that nurses score higher on depression scales when they start working the night shift (Smith et al. 1982). Retired shift workers also have a higher rate of depression compared with retired day workers (Scott 2000). Because regular schedules can assist in the therapy of mania, patients with bipolar disorder may be at particular risk for the adverse consequences of shift work (Reynolds et al. 1995).

Treatment

The goal of clinical management is to align the circadian propensity for sleep and wakefulness with the work schedule, as well as to employ behavioral approaches to improve sleep quality and work performance. For rotating shifts, a clockwise rotation, in which the schedule is delayed from day to evening to night, is recommended. Because disturbances in sleep and wakefulness are most common among night shift workers, most of the specific strategies have focused on this group.

In night shift workers, timed bright light and melatonin have been shown to accelerate circadian adaptation (Burgess et al. 2002; Dawson and Campbell 1991; Dawson et al. 1995; Sharkey et al. 2001). Various light intensities, from 1,200 to 10,000 lux, with duration of exposure ranging from 3 to 6 hours, have been used successfully to realign circadian rhythms and improve performance during the night shift (Burgess et al. 2002). Recently, a regimen of intermittent exposure to bright light (20-minute per hour blocks) during the night shift has also been shown to accelerate adaptation to shift work (Boivin and James 2002). It is recommended that either intermittent or continuous light exposure begin early in the shift and terminate approximately 2 hours before the end of the shift to avoid the potential delaying effects of early morning bright light (Crowley et al. 2003). Exposure to bright light during the commute home has been shown to prevent this necessary phase delay, with the result that the circadian sleep propensity rhythm will not align with the desired sleep time. Several studies have shown that avoiding this bright light exposure in the morning may be just as important as increasing exposure to light during the night shift (Boivin and James 2002; Crowley et al. 2003). A few studies have shown that after a night shift melatonin given at bedtime was effective at increasing sleep duration but had limited effects on alertness (Burgess et al. 2002).

It is unclear whether improvements in sleep were due to the hypnotic or the phase-resetting properties of melatonin. Furthermore, melatonin has not been shown to provide additional benefits when combined with a regimen of intermittent bright light therapy and morning light avoidance (Crowley et al. 2003).

In addition to circadian alignment, pharmacologic agents can be used to improve sleep quality and alertness. Hypnotic medications may be used to treat insomnia, but they do not necessarily address the circadian misalignment and therefore are often insufficient, particularly in the management of excessive sleepiness. Caffeine use has been shown to be an effective short-term strategy to alleviate excessive sleepiness, one of the most debilitating symptoms of this disorder (Babkoff et al. 2002). More recently, the U.S. Food and Drug Administration (FDA) has approved modafinil for the treatment of excessive sleepiness associated with shift work. A recent trial found that 200 mg of modafinil given at the start of a night shift reduced subsequent sleepiness and neurobehavioral deficits (Walsh et al. 2004).

It is important to recognize that family, social, and environmental factors are very important in the successful management of shift work–related sleep and wake disturbances. Family responsibilities such as household chores and child care can limit time available for sleep, and marital dynamics can affect ability to cope with shift work. Adherence to good sleep habits and practices is a basic approach for all patients. Careful attention to protect and improve the sleep environment by decreasing daytime noise and providing a dark and comfortable room is important. Education of the individual, family, and employer regarding the need to protect sleep time and (when appropriate) to provide strategies at work to improve performance and safety is essential for effective management of this disorder.

Jet Lag Syndrome

(In DSM-IV-TR, the pertinent classification is *circadian rhythm sleep disorder, jet lag type*. In ICSD-2, it is *time zone change [jet lag] type*.)

The sleep-wake disturbance associated with jet lag occurs with rapid travel across time zones, resulting in a transient alteration between the external physical environment and the timing of the endogenous circadian rhythm. Symptoms typically include difficulty falling asleep at night, daytime sleepiness, general malaise, gastrointestinal upset, and mood changes (Winget et al. 1984). Circadian and sleep disruption due to jet lag may exacerbate affective disorders (Katz et al. 2002). Symptoms are transient (in contrast to those in shift work type) and resolve as the traveler adjusts to the new time zone.

Although there are substantial interindividual differences in the severity of jet lag symptoms, the two major factors that influence the severity and duration of symptoms are the direction of travel and the number of time zones crossed. Eastward travel, in which adjustment requires an advance shift of circadian rhythms, is usually more difficult than westward travel (Wagner 1996). Up to 80% of business travelers have difficulty with sleep following eastward travel (Wagner 1996). However, travel in both directions can result in sleep disturbances. With eastward travel, sleep-onset difficulties are more common, whereas with westward travel, sleep maintenance problems are more prominent (Boulos et al. 1995). Other factors, such as poor air quality, lack of physical activity, and dehydration also contribute to sleep loss and the malaise that often accompany jet travel.

Treatment of jet lag needs to address both reentrainment of the circadian clock and sleep loss. Travelers should be encouraged to wear loose, comfortable clothing, use ear plugs and eyeshades, and increase fluid intake, but to avoid excessive alcohol and caffeinated beverages during the flight. On arrival, eating meals at local times, getting exercise and light exposure at appropriate times, and maintaining good sleep habits can ameliorate jet lag symptoms and improve nighttime sleep (Waterhouse et al. 1997).

Approaches to accelerate circadian entrainment to the new time zone include appropriately timed bright light exposure, avoidance of light exposure at the wrong time of the day (Burgess et al. 2003), and use of melatonin (Beaumont et al. 2004; Burgess et al. 2003). The timing of light exposure is dependent on the direction of travel. For example, on eastward flights travelers should stay awake upon arrival but avoid bright light in the early morning and try to get light in the afternoon (Herxheimer and Waterhouse 2003).

Several studies have also shown that treatment with melatonin 2–5 mg close to local bedtime for up to 4 days can alleviate jet lag (Herxheimer and Petrie 2002; Herxheimer and Waterhouse 2003). As mentioned in previous sections, melatonin is available as a nutritional supplement, but it has not been approved by the FDA for the treatment of CRSDs. In addition to circadian strategies, short-term use of a short-acting hypnotic agent is also useful in the management of insomnia symptoms with jet lag. Zolpidem taken after arrival for 3 nights at bedtime has been shown to be an effective method for reducing sleep disturbance after travel (Jamieson et al. 2001).

Summary

Circadian rhythm sleep disorders should be considered in the evaluation of all patients who present with complaints of insomnia or excessive sleepiness. Circadian rhythm disorders, specifically in patients with DSPT and ASPT, may be comorbid with personality and mood disorders. Because of the limited availability of practical diagnostic tools and the lack of large-scale randomized controlled clinical trials, evaluation and treatment of CRSDs remain challenging.

References

Akerstedt T: [Increased risk of accidents during night shift: an underestimated problem are fatigue-induced accidents] (Swedish). Lakartidningen 92:2103–2104, 1995

Akerstedt T: Shift work and disturbed sleep-wakefulness. Occup Med (Lond) 53:89–94, 2003

Alvarez B, Dahlitz MJ, Vignau J, et al: The delayed sleep phase syndrome: clinical and investigative findings in 14 subjects. J Neurol Neurosurg Psychiatry 55:665–670, 1992

American Academy of Sleep Medicine: The International Classification of Sleep Disorders, 2nd Edition. Westchester, IL, American Academy of Sleep Medicine (in press)

American Psychiatric Association: Diagnostic and Statistical Manual of Mental Disorders, 4th Edition, Text Revision. Washington, DC, American Psychiatric Association, 2000

Ancoli-Israel S, Kripke DK: Prevalent sleep problems in the aged. Biofeedback Self Regul 16:349–359, 1991

Ancoli-Israel S, Schnierow B, Kelsoe J, et al: A pedigree of one family with delayed sleep phase syndrome. Chronobiol Int 18:831–840, 2001

Ancoli-Israel S, Martin JL, Kripke DF, et al: Effect of light treatment on sleep and circadian rhythms in demented nursing home patients. J Am Geriatr Soc 50:282–289, 2002

Ando K, Kripke DF, Ancoli-Israel S, et al: Estimated prevalence of delayed and advanced sleep phase syndromes. Sleep Res 24:509, 1995

Aoki H, Ozeki Y, Yamada N, et al: Hypersensitivity of melatonin suppression in response to light in patients with delayed sleep phase syndrome. Chronobiol Int 18: 263–271, 2001

Archer SN, Robilliard DL, Skene DJ, et al: A length polymorphism in the circadian clock gene Per3 is linked to delayed sleep phase syndrome and extreme diurnal preference. Sleep 26:413–415, 2003

Aschoff J, Fatranska M, Giedke H, et al: Human circadian rhythms in continuous darkness: entrainment by social cues. Science 171:213–215, 1971

Babkoff H, French J, Whitmore J, et al: Single-dose bright light and/or caffeine effect on nocturnal performance. Aviat Space Environ Med 73:341–350, 2002

Baehr EK, Eastman CI, Revelle W, et al: Circadian phase-shifting effects of nocturnal exercise in older compared to young adults. Am J Physiol Regul Integr Comp Physiol 284:R1542–R1550, 2003

Beaumont M, Batejat D, Pierard C, et al: Caffeine or melatonin effects on sleep and sleepiness after rapid eastward transmeridian travel. J Appl Physiol 96:50–58, 2004

Bellingham J, Foster RG: Opsins and mammalian photoentrainment. Cell Tissue Res 309:57–71, 2002

Berk ML, Finkelstein JA: An autoradiographic determination of the efferent projections of the suprachiasmatic nucleus of the hypothalamus. Brain Res 226:1–13, 1981

Boivin DB, James FO: Circadian adaptation to night-shift work by judicious light and darkness exposure. J Biol Rhythms 17:556–567, 2002

Boivin DB, Duffy JF, Kronauer RE, et al: Sensitivity of the human circadian pacemaker to moderately bright light. J Biol Rhythms 9:315–331, 1994

Boulos Z, Campbell SS, Lewy AJ, et al: Light treatment for sleep disorders: consensus report, VII: jet lag. J Biol Rhythms 10:167–176, 1995

Burgess HJ, Sharkey KM, Eastman CI: Bright light, dark and melatonin can promote circadian adaptation in night shift workers. Sleep Med Rev 6: 407–420, 2002

Burgess HJ, Crowley SJ, Gazda CJ, et al: Preflight adjustment to eastward travel: 3 days of advancing sleep with and without morning bright light. J Biol Rhythms 18:318–328, 2003

Buxton OM, Frank SA, L'Hermite-Baleriaux M, et al: Roles of intensity and duration of nocturnal exercise in causing phase delays of human circadian rhythms. Am J Physiol 273:E536–E542, 1997

Cajochen C, Krauchi K, Wirz-Justice A: Role of melatonin in the regulation of human circadian rhythms and sleep. J Neuroendocrinol 15:432–437, 2003

Campbell SS: Intrinsic disruption of normal sleep and circadian patterns, in Regulation of Sleep and Circadian Rhythms, Vol 133. Edited by Turek FW, Zee PC. New York, Marcel Dekker, 1999, pp 465–486

Carskadon M, Dement W: Sleep studies on a 90-minute day. Electroencephalogr Clin Neurophysiol 39:145–155, 1975

Carskadon M, Dement W: Sleep tendency: an objective measure of sleep loss. Sleep Res 6:200–201, 1977

Carskadon MA, Labyak SE, Acebo C, et al: Intrinsic circadian period of adolescent humans measured in conditions of forced desynchrony. Neurosci Lett 260:129–132, 1999

Chesson AL Jr, Littner M, Davila D, et al: Practice parameters for the use of light therapy in the treatment of sleep disorders. Standards of Practice Committee, American Academy of Sleep Medicine. Sleep 22:641–660, 1999

Crowley SJ, Lee C, Tseng CY, et al: Combinations of bright light, scheduled dark, sunglasses, and melatonin to facilitate circadian entrainment to night shift work. J Biol Rhythms 18:513–523, 2003

Czeisler CA, Weitzman E, Moore-Ede MC, et al: Human sleep: its duration and organization depend on its circadian phase. Science 210:1264–1267, 1980

Czeisler CA, Allan JS, Strogatz SH, et al: Bright light resets the human circadian pacemaker independent of the timing of the sleep-wake cycle. Science 233:667–671, 1986

Czeisler CA, Shanahan TL, Klerman EB, et al: Suppression of melatonin secretion in some blind patients by exposure to bright light. N Engl J Med 332:6–11, 1995

Czeisler CA, Duffy JF, Shanahan TL, et al: Stability, precision, and near-24-hour period of the human circadian pacemaker. Science 284:2177–2181, 1999

Dagan Y: Circadian rhythm sleep disorders (CRSD). Sleep Med Rev 6:45–54, 2002

Dagan Y, Sela H, Omer H, et al: High prevalence of personality disorders among circadian rhythm sleep disorders (CRSD) patients. J Psychosom Res 41:357–363, 1996

Dagan Y, Stein D, Steinbock M, et al: Frequency of delayed sleep phase syndrome among hospitalized adolescent psychiatric patients. J Psychosom Res 45:15–20, 1998

Dagan Y: Circadian rhythm sleep disorders (CRSD). Sleep Med Rev 6:45–54, 2002

Dahlitz M, Alvarez B, Vignau J, et al: Delayed sleep phase syndrome response to melatonin. Lancet 337:1121–1124, 1991

Dantz B, Edgar DM, Dement WC: Circadian rhythms in narcolepsy: studies on a 90 minute day. Electroencephalogr Clin Neurophysiol 90:24–35, 1994

Dawson D, Campbell SS: Timed exposure to bright light improves sleep and alertness during simulated night shifts. Sleep 14:511–516, 1991

Dawson D, Encel N, Lushington K: Improving adaptation to simulated night shift: timed exposure to bright light versus daytime melatonin administration. Sleep 18:11–21, 1995

Dijk DJ, Czeisler CA: Paradoxical timing of the circadian rhythm of sleep propensity serves to consolidate sleep and wakefulness in humans. Neurosci Lett 166:63–68, 1994

Dijk DJ, Czeisler CA: Contribution of the circadian pacemaker and the sleep homeostat to sleep propensity, sleep structure, electroencephalographic slow waves, and sleep spindle activity in humans. J Neurosci 15:3526–3528, 1995

Duffy JF, Czeisler CA: Age-related change in the relationship between circadian period, circadian phase, and diurnal preference in humans. Neurosci Lett 318: 117–120, 2002

Dumont M, Benhaberou-Brun D, Paquet J, et al: Profile of 24-h light exposure and circadian phase of melatonin secretion in night workers. J Biol Rhythms 16:502–511, 2001

Dunlap JC: Molecular bases for circadian clocks. Cell 96:271–290, 1999

Ebisawa T, Uchiyama M, Kajimura N, et al: Association of structural polymorphisms in the human period3 gene with delayed sleep phase syndrome. EMBO Rep 2:342–346, 2001

Guido ME, Carpentieri AR, Gabarino-Pico E: Circadian phototransduction and the regulation of biological rhythms. Neurochem Res 27:1473–1489, 2002

Herxheimer A, Petrie KJ: Melatonin for the prevention and treatment of jet lag. Cochrane Database Syst Rev (2):CD001520, 2002

Herxheimer A, Waterhouse J: The prevention and treatment of jet lag. BMJ 326:296–297, 2003

Hohjoh H, Takasu M, Shishsikura K, et al: Significant association of the arylalkylamine N-acetyltransferase (AA-NAT) gene with delayed sleep phase syndrome. Neurogenetics 4:151–153, 2003

Hoogendijk WJ, van Someren EJ, Mirmiran M, et al: Circadian rhythm-related behavioral disturbances and structural hypothalamic changes in Alzheimer's disease. Int Psychogeriatr 8 (suppl 3):245–252, 1996

Horne JA, Ostberg O: A self-assessment questionnaire to determine morningness-eveningness in human circadian rhythms. Int J Chronobiol 4:97–110, 1976

Iwase T, Kajimura N, Uchiyama M, et al: Mutation screening of the human Clock gene in circadian rhythm sleep disorders. Psychiatry Res 109:121–128, 2002

Jamieson AO, Zammit GK, Rosenberg RS, et al: Zolpidem reduces the sleep disturbance of jet lag. Sleep Med 2:423–430, 2001

Jones CR, Campbell SS, Zone SE, et al: Familial advanced sleep-phase syndrome: a short-period circadian rhythm variant in humans. Nat Med 5:1062–1065, 1999

Kamei Y, Urata J, Uchiyaya M, et al: Clinical characteristics of circadian rhythm sleep disorders. Psychiatry Clin Neurosci 52:234–235, 1998

Kamgar-Parsi B, Wehr TA, Gillin JC, et al: Successful treatment of human non-24-hour sleep-wake syndrome. Sleep 6:257–264, 1983

Katz G, Knobler HY, Laibel Z, et al: Time zone change and major psychiatric morbidity: the results of a 6-year study in Jerusalem. Compr Psychiatry 43:37–40, 2002

Knauth P, Landau K, Droge C, et al: Duration of sleep depending on the type of shift work. Int Arch Occup Environ Health 4:167–177, 1980

Lack L, Schumacher K: Evening light treatment of early morning insomnia. Sleep Res 22:225–227, 1993

Lewy AJ, Bauer VK, Cutler NL, et al: Morning vs evening light treatment of patients with winter depression. Arch Gen Psychiatry 55:890–896, 1998

Lewy AJ, Bauer VK, Hasler BP, et al: Capturing the circadian rhythms of free-running blind people with 0.5 mg melatonin. Brain Res 918:96–100, 2001

Littner MR, Kushida C, Wise M, et al: Practice parameters for clinical use of the multiple sleep latency test and the maintenance of wakefulness test. Sleep 28:113–121

Lockley SW, Brainard GC, Czeisler CA: High sensitivity of the human circadian melatonin rhythm to resetting by short wavelength light. J Clin Endocrinol Metab 88:4502–4505, 2003

McArthur AJ, Lewy AJ, Sack RL: Non-24-hour sleep-wake syndrome in a sighted man: circadian rhythm studies and efficacy of melatonin treatment. Sleep 19:544–553, 1996

Menaker M: Circadian rhythms: circadian photoreception. Science 299:213–214, 2003

Miles LE, Raynal DM, Wilson MA: Blind man living in normal society has circadian rhythms of 24.9 hours. Science 198:421–423, 1977

Minors DS, Waterhouse JM, Wirz-Justice A: A human phase-response curve to light. Neurosci Lett 133:36–40, 1991

Miyamoto Y, Sancar A: Vitamin B_2-based blue-light photoreceptors in the retinohypothalamic tract as the photoactive pigments for setting the circadian clock in mammals. Proc Natl Acad Sci U S A 95:6097–6102, 1998

Moldofsky H, Musisi S, Phillipson EA: Treatment of a case of advanced sleep phase syndrome by phase advance chronotherapy. Sleep 9:61–65, 1986

Moore RY: Circadian rhythms: basic neurobiology and clinical applications. Annu Rev Med 48:253–266, 1997

Moore RY: A clock for the ages. Science 284:2102–2103, 1999

Moore RY, Eichler VB: Loss of a circadian adrenal corticosterone rhythm following suprachiasmatic lesions in the rat. Brain Res 42:201–206, 1972

Nagtegaal JE, Laurant MW, Kerkhof GA, et al: Effects of melatonin on the quality of life in patients with delayed sleep phase syndrome. J Psychosom Res 48:45–50, 2000

Naylor E, Penev PD, Orbeta L, et al: Daily social and physical activity increases slow-wave sleep and daytime neuropsychological performance in the elderly. Sleep 23:87–95, 2000

Ohta T, Iwata T, Kayukawa Y, et al: Daily activity and persistent sleep-wake schedule disorders. Prog Neuropsychopharmacol Biol Psychiatry 16:529–537, 1992

Okawa M, Mishima K, Hishikawa Y, et al: Circadian rhythm disorders in sleep-waking and body temperature in elderly patients with dementia and their treatment. Sleep 14:478–485, 1991

Oldani A, Ferini-Strambi L, Zucconi M, et al: Melatonin and delayed sleep phase syndrome: ambulatory polygraphic evaluation. Neuroreport 6:132–134, 1994

Oren DA, Wehr TA: Hypernyctohemeral syndrome after chronotherapy for delayed sleep phase syndrome (letter). N Engl J Med 327:1762, 1992

Ozaki N, Iwata T, Itoh A, et al: A treatment trial of delayed sleep phase syndrome with triazolam. Jpn J Psychiatry Neurol 43:51–55, 1989

Ozaki S, Uchiyama M, Shirakawa S, et al: Prolonged interval from body temperature nadir to sleep offset in patients with delayed sleep phase syndrome. Sleep 19:36–40, 1996

Palm L, Blennow G, Wetterberg L: Long-term melatonin treatment in blind children and young adults with circadian sleep-wake disturbances. Dev Med Child Neurol 39:319–325, 1997

Pelayo R, Thorpy MJ, Govinsky P, et al: Prevalence of delayed sleep phase syndrome among adolescents. Sleep Res 17:392–393, 1988

Pillar G, Shahar E, Peled N, et al: Melatonin improves sleep-wake patterns in psychomotor retarded children. Pediatr Neurol 23:225–228, 2000

Pollak CP, Stokes PE: Circadian rest-activity rhythms in demented and nondemented older community residents and their caregivers. J Am Geriatr Soc 45:446–452, 1997

Presser HB: Towards a 24 hour economy. Science 284:1778–1779, 1999

Ralph MR, Menaker M: A mutation of the circadian system in golden hamsters. Science 241:1225–1227, 1988

Regestein QR, Monk TH: Delayed sleep phase syndrome: a review of its clinical aspects. Am J Psychiatry 152:602–608, 1995

Regestein QR, Pavlova M: Treatment of delayed sleep phase syndrome. Gen Hosp Psychiatry 17:335–345, 1995

Reid KJ, Chang AM, Dubocovich ML, et al: Familial advanced sleep phase syndrome. Arch Neurol 58:1089–1094, 2001

Reinberg A, Motohashi Y, Bourdeleau P, et al: Internal desynchronization of circadian rhythms and tolerance of shift work. Chronobiologia 16:21–34, 1989

Reynolds CF 3rd, Frank E, Perel JM, et al: Maintenance therapies for late-life recurrent major depression: research and review circa 1995. Int Psychogeriatr 7(suppl):27–39, 1995

Rosenthal NE, Joseph-Vanderpool JR, Levendosky AA, et al: Phase-shifting effects of bright morning light as treatment for delayed sleep phase syndrome. Sleep 13:354–361, 1990

Sack RL, Lewy AJ: Circadian rhythm sleep disorders: lessons from the blind. Sleep Med Rev 5:189–206, 2001

Sack RL, Lewy AJ, Blood ML, et al: Circadian rhythm abnormalities in totally blind people: incidence and clinical significance. J Clin Endocrinol Metab 75:127–134, 1992

Sack RL, Brandes RW, Kendall AR, et al: Entrainment of free-running circadian rhythms by melatonin in blind people. N Engl J Med 343:1070–1077, 2000

Salin-Pascual RJ, Granados Fuentes D, Nieto Caraveo A: [Syndrome of delayed phase sleep: report of 3 cases] (Spanish). Rev Invest Clin 40:405–412, 1988

Satoh K, Mishima K, Inouye Y, et al: Two pedigrees of familial advanced sleep phase syndrome in Japan. Sleep 26:416–417, 2003

Schnelle JF, Cruise PA, Alessi CA, et al: Sleep hygiene in physically dependent nursing home residents: behavioral and environmental intervention implications. Sleep 21:515–523, 1998

Schrader H, Bovim G, Sand T: Depression in the delayed sleep phase syndrome (letter). Am J Psychiatry 153:1238, 1996

Scott AJ: Shift work and health. Prim Care 27:1057–1079, 2000

Sharkey KM, Fogg LF, Eastman CI: Effects of melatonin administration on daytime sleep after simulated night shift work. J Sleep Res 10:181–192, 2001

Shirayama M, Shirayama Y, Iida H, et al: The psychological aspects of patients with delayed sleep phase syndrome (DSPS). Sleep Med 4:427–433, 2003

Smith MJ, Colligan MJ, Tasto DL: Health and safety consequences of shift work in the food processing industry. Ergonomics 25:133–144, 1982

Stephan FK, Zucker I: Circadian rhythms in drinking behavior and locomotor activity of rats are eliminated by hypothalamic lesions. Proc Natl Acad Sci U S A 69:1583–1586, 1972

Strogatz SH, Kronauer RE, Czeisler CA: Circadian pacemaker interferes with sleep onset at specific times each day: role in insomnia. Am J Physiol 253 (1 pt 2):R172–R178, 1987

Takahashi Y, Hohjoh H, Maatsuura K: Predisposing factors in delayed sleep phase syndrome. Psychiatry Clin Neurosci 54:356–358, 2000

Thorpy MJ, Korman E, Spielman AJ, et al: Delayed sleep phase syndrome in adolescents. J Adolesc Health Care 9:22–27, 1988

Toh KL, Jones CR, He Y, et al: An hPer2 phosphorylation site mutation in familial advanced sleep phase syndrome. Science 291:1040–1043, 2001

Uchiyama M, Okawa M, Shirakawa S, et al: A polysomnographic study on patients with delayed sleep phase syndrome (DSPS). Jpn J Psychiatry Neurol 46:219–221, 1992

Uchiyama M, Okawa M, Shibui K, et al: Poor recovery sleep after sleep deprivation in delayed sleep phase syndrome. Psychiatry Clin Neurosci 53:195–197, 1999

Uchiyama M, Okawa M, Shibui K, et al: Poor compensatory function for sleep loss as a pathogenic factor in patients with delayed sleep phase syndrome. Sleep 23:553–558, 2000

Uchiyama M, Shibui K, Hayakawa T, et al: Larger phase angle between sleep propensity and melatonin rhythms in sighted humans with non-24-hour sleep-wake syndrome. Sleep 25:83–88, 2002

Van Someren EJ, Hagebeuk EE, Lijzenga C, et al: Circadian rest-activity rhythm disturbances in Alzheimer's disease. Biol Psychiatry 40:259–270, 1996

Van Someren EJ, Swaab DF, Colenda CC, et al: Bright light therapy: improved sensitivity to its effects on rest-activity rhythms in Alzheimer patients by application of nonparametric methods. Chronobiol Int 16:505–518, 1999

Vitaterna MH, King DP, Chang AM, et al: Mutagenesis and mapping of a mouse gene, Clock, essential for circadian behavior. Science 264:719–725, 1994

Wagner DR: Disorders of the circadian sleep-wake cycle. Neurol Clin 14:651–670, 1996

Walsh JK, Randazzo AC, Stone KL, et al: Modafinil improves alertness, vigilance, and executive function during simulated night shifts. Sleep 27:434–439, 2004

Warman VL, Dijk DJ, Warman GR, et al: Phase advancing human circadian rhythms with short wavelength light. Neurosci Lett 342:37–40, 2003

Waterhouse J, Reilly T, Atkinson G: Jet-lag. Lancet 350:1611–1616, 1997

Weitzman ED, Czeisler CA, Coleman RM, et al: Delayed sleep phase syndrome: a chronobiological disorder with sleep-onset insomnia. Arch Gen Psychiatry 38:737–746, 1981

Winget CM, DeRoshia CW, Markley CL, et al: A review of human physiological and performance changes associated with desynchronosis of biological rhythms. Aviat Space Environ Med 55:1085–1096, 1984

Witting W, Kwa IH, Eikelenboom P, et al: Alterations in the circadian rest-activity rhythm in aging and Alzheimer's disease. Biol Psychiatry 27:563–572, 1990

Yamadera H, Takahashi K, Okawa M: A multicenter study of sleep-wake rhythm disorders: clinical features of sleep-wake rhythm disorders. Psychiatry Clin Neurosci 50:195–201, 1996

Zeitzer JM, Dijk DJ, Kronaure R, et al: Sensitivity of the human circadian pacemaker to nocturnal light: melatonin phase resetting and suppression. J Physiol 526:695–702, 2000

Zheng B, Larkin DW, Albrecht U, et al: The mPer2 gene encodes a functional component of the mammalian circadian clock. Nature 400: 169–173, 1999

Zulley J, Wever R, Aschoff J: The dependence of onset and duration of sleep on the circadian rhythm of rectal temperature. Pflugers Arch 391:314–318, 1981

Index

*Page numbers printed in **boldface** type refer to tables or figures.*

Elderly *(continued)*
  side effects of benzodiazepines in,
    54
Electrocardiograms (EEGs)
  hyperarousal in insomnia and, 33
  hypnograms in healthy subjects
    and, **10–11**
  polysomnography and, 5
Electroencephalogram (EEG)
  confusional arousals in
    parasomnias and, 166
  ventilatory effort in sleep apnea
    and, 78, **79**
Electromyographic (EMG) recording,
    and polysomnography, 5
Electrooculographic (EOG)
    recording, and
    polysomnography, 5
Electrophysiology, and hyperarousal
    in insomnia, 33
Emotional processing, role of sleep
    in, 2
Emotions, as trigger for cataplexy, 111
Encephalitis, and excessive daytime
    sleepiness, 119
Endocrine disorders, and insomnia,
    38. *See also* Neuroendrocrinology
Endogenous circadian rhythms, 3–4
Entrainment, of circadian rhythms, 3,
    186
Environmental advantage, and
    theories of function of sleep, 1–2
Epidemiology. *See also* Prevalence
  of advanced sleep phase type of
    circadian rhythm disorder,
    198
  confusional arousals in
    parasomnia and, 164
  of delayed sleep phase type of
    circadian rhythm disorder,
    193
  of excessive daytime sleepiness,
    108–109
  of insomnia, 30–32

of irregular sleep-wake type of
    circadian rhythm disorder,
    204–205
  of narcolepsy, 112
  of nonentrained type of circadian
    rhythm disorder, 201
  of shift work type of circadian
    rhythm disorder, 206–207
  of sleep apnea, 81–82
Epilepsy
  excessive daytime sleepiness and,
    119
  gabapentin and insomnia in, 63
Epworth Sleepiness Scale (ESS), 15,
    88, 100
Eszopiclone, and insomnia, **52,** 53
Ethnicity, and prevalence of restless
    legs syndrome, 145. *See also*
    African Americans
Etiology
  of advanced sleep phase type of
    circadian rhythm disorder, 199
  of delayed sleep phase type of
    circadian rhythm disorder,
    193–194
  of insomnia, 32–37
Etiology-based classifications, of
    insomnia, 41–42
Evolution, and theories of function of
    sleep, 1
Excessive daytime sleepiness (EDS)
  comorbid disorders of
    somnolence and, 108
  delayed sleep phase type of
    circadian rhythm disorder
    and, 191, 193
  epidemiology of, 108–109
  insufficient sleep and primary
    syndromes of, 109–120
  management of, 120–123
  multiple sleep latency test (MSLT)
    and, 19
  nervous system disorders and,
    118–120

sleep apnea and, **85,** 87, **88,** 99
Excessive sleep inertia. *See* Sleep drunkenness
Experience, sleep and integration of, 2

Falls, and side effects of benzodiazepines, 54
Family, and shift work–related sleep, 209
Family history. *See also* Genetics
of idiopathic hypersomnia, 115
of restless legs syndrome, 147
Fatigue, and sleep apnea, 98–99
Fear, of loss of sleep, 47
Fibromyalgia, and insomnia, **38**
Flumazenil, and idiopathic recurring stupor, 118
Fluoxetine, and zolpidem as adjunctive medication, 56
Flurazepam, **52**
Fluvoxamine, and delayed sleep phase type of circadian rhythm disorder, 195–196
Fragmented sleep
excessive daytime sleepiness and, 109
narcolepsy and, 112
Free-running period, of circadian rhythmn, 186
Functional neuroanatomic studies, of hyperarousal and insomnia, 33–34

Gabapentin
insomnia and, **59,** 62–63, 64
restless legs syndrome and, **154,** 155, 156
GABA receptor complex
benzodiazepine receptor agonists and, 50–51
tigabine and, 63
valerian and, 62

Gastroesophageal reflux, and insomnia, **38**
Gastrointestinal disease, and insomnia, **38**
Gender. *See* Men; Women
Genetics. *See also* Family history
advanced sleep phase type of circadian rhythm disorder and, 199
circadian rhythms and, 186
confusional arousals in parasomnia and, 164, 166
of delayed sleep phase type of circadian rhythm disorder, 193
of narcolepsy, 125–130
of restless legs syndrome, 147
sleep terrors and, 169
of sleepwalking, 167
variations in circadian rhythms and, 4–5
Graphic sleep diary, **16**

Hallucinations, and narcolepsy, 112
Head trauma, and excessive daytime sleepiness, 119
Health, relationship between sleep and, 2–3
Heart failure, and sleep apnea, 89. *See also* Cardiovascular disease; Congestive heart failure
Heuristic model, of insomnia, **36**
Hip fractures, and side effects of benzodiazepines, 54
Histamine, and wakefulness, 60, 129
Histocompatibility human leukocyte antigen (HLA) testing, for narcolepsy, 114
Homeostatic factors, in physiological regulation of sleep, 11–13
Horne-Ostberg questionnaire, 191
Human leukocyte antigen (HLA), and narcolepsy, 124–125
Humidifiers, and sleep apnea, 93

Modafinil *(continued)*
  sleep apnea and, 100
Monoamine oxidase inhibitors
  (MAOIs), and REM sleep
  behavior disorder, 176
Mood disorders, and shift work type
  of circadian rhythm disorder,
  207–208
Mortality, association between sleep
  duration and, 2
Motor restlessness, and restless legs
  syndrome, 149
Motor vehicles. *See* Accidents
Multiple sleep latency test (MSLT),
  19, 113, 207
Muscle tone, and cataplexy, 111
Myocardial infarction, and sleep
  apnea, **85**
Myotonic dystrophy, and excessive
  daytime sleepiness, 119

Naps, and management of excessive
  daytime sleepiness, 120
Narcolepsy
  features of compared to idiopathic
    hypersomnia, **116**
  hypocretin transmission in canine
    and human, 125–130
  misunderstanding and
    misdiagnosis of, 108
  pathophysiology of, 123–125
  prevalence of, 109
  as primary disorder of excessive
    daytime sleepiness, 110–114
Nasal congestion, and sleep apnea,
  92–93
National Institutes of Health, 140
Natural history, of insomnia, 31–32
Neurobiology, of circadian rhythms,
  3–5, 185–190
Neurocognitive complications, of
  sleep apnea, **85,** 87–89
Neurocognitive model, of insomnia,
  36

Neurodegenerative disorders, and
  excessive daytime sleepiness or
  sleep disruption, 119
Neuroendrocrinology, and
  hyperarousal in insomnia, 33.
  See also Endocrine disorders
Neurological disorders. *See also*
  Central nervous system
  excessive daytime sleepiness and,
    118–120
  insomnia and, **38**
  REM sleep behavior disorder and,
    176
  restless legs syndrome and, 150
Neuromuscular disorders, and
  excessive daytime sleepiness,
  119
Neuropathy
  excessive daytime sleepiness and,
    119
  insomnia and, **38**
  restless legs syndrome and, 149
Neuropsychological function, and
  sleep apnea, **85**
Neurotransmitters, and regulation of
  sleep-wake cycles, 14. *See also*
  Dopamine system
Nicotine, and insomnia, **39**
Night, and worsening of restless legs
  syndrome, 143
Nightmare disorder, **165,** 177–178
Nocturnal dysrhythmias, and sleep
  apnea, **85**
Nocturnal eating syndrome, 172–173
Nocturnal hypoxemia, and sleep
  apnea, 89
Nocturnal leg cramps, and restless
  legs syndrome, 149
Nonentrained type, of circadian
  rhythm disorder, **192,** 201–204
Non-REM parasomnias, 163–173, **174**
Non-REM sleep
  brain regions and generation of,
    13–14

classification of disorders of
arousal and, **24**
definition and characteristics of, 5
examples of polysomnographic
patterns of, **6–8**
PET study of primary insomnia
and, 33–34, **35**
Norepinephrine, and narcolepsy, 129
Nottingham Health Profile, 88

Obesity, and sleep apnea, 91. *See also*
Body weight
Obstructive sleep apnea/hypopnea
syndrome (OSAH). *See* Sleep
apnea
Olanzapine, and insomnia, **59,** 63–64
Opioids, and restless legs syndrome,
154, 155
Optimizing waking function, and
theories of function of sleep, 2
Oral appliance therapy, and sleep
apnea, 93–95
Orexin. *See* Hypocretin
Osteoarthritis, and insomnia, **38**
Oxycodone, and restless legs
syndrome, **154,** 155

Palatal surgery, for sleep apnea, 97
Panic attacks, and sleep terrors, 170
Paradoxical intention, and insomnia, 47
Parasomnias. *See also* Confusional
arousals; Nightmare disorder;
REM sleep behavior disorder;
Sleep-related eating disorder;
Sleep terrors; Sleepwalking
classification of sleep disorders
and, **21, 24–25**
definition of, 19, 163
in non-REM sleep, 163–173
overview of, **165**
pharmacologic treatment of, **174–
175**
polysomnography and evaluation
of, 19

in REM sleep, 173, **175,** 176–178
Parkinson's disease
insomnia and, **38**
REM sleep behavior disorder and,
176
Pathophysiology and pathogenesis
of advanced sleep phase type of
circadian rhythm disorder, 199
of delayed sleep phase type of
circadian rhythm disorder,
193–194
of insomnia, 32–37
of irregular sleep-wake type of
circadian rhythm disorder, 205
of narcolepsy, 123–125
of nonentrained type of circadian
rhythm disorder, 202–203
of restless legs syndrome, 146–149
of shift work type of circadian
rhythm disorder, 207
of sleep apnea, 82–84
Patient history
clinical assessment of insomnia
and, 37, 40
clinical assessment of sleep and
circadian rhythm disorders
and, 14–15
sleep apnea and, **90**
Pemoline, and excessive daytime
sleepiness, **121**
Pergolide, and restless legs
syndrome, **154,** 155
Periodic limb movements of sleep
(PLMS), 143–144, **145**
Personality disorders, and circadian
rhythm disorders, 193, 203
Pharmacology. *See also* Adjunctive
medications; Anticonvulsants;
Antidepressants;
Antipsychotics;
Benzodiazepines; Hypnotics;
Selective serotonin reuptake
inhibitors; Side effects;
Stimulants; Tolerance; Treatment

growth in field of, 20–21
overview of clinical assessment of, 14–20
types of, 19–20
Sleep disorders related to another mental disorder, **21**
Sleep disorders related to general medical conditions, **21**
Sleep drive, and duration of wakefulness, **12,** 13
Sleep drunkenness
confusional arousals and, 166
idiopathic hypersomnia and, 116
Sleep duration, association between mortality and, 2
Sleep Heart Health Study, 79
Sleep histogram. *See* Hypnogram
Sleep hygiene
insomnia and, **46,** 47
shift work-related sleep and, 209
Sleep logs. *See* Actigraphy
Sleep-onset REM periods (SOREMPs), and narcolepsy, 113
Sleep paralysis, and narcolepsy, 112
Sleep regulation, two-process model of, 11–13
Sleep-related abnormal sexual behavior, 166
Sleep-related breathing disorders, and classification of sleep disorders, **22–23**
Sleep-related eating disorder (SRED), **165,** 171–173, **174**
Sleep-related hypoventilation/ hypoxemic syndromes, **22–23**
Sleep-related movement disorders, and classification of sleep disorders, **25**
Sleep-related violence, 166–167
Sleep restriction therapy, for insomnia, 43, **45,** 47–48
Sleep terrors, **165,** 169–170, 177
Sleep-wake cycles. *See also* Circadian rhythms; Wakefulness

clinical assessment and regularity and timing of, 15
major theories of function of, 1–3
neurotransmitters and regulation of, 14
Sleep-wake diaries
clinical assessment of sleep disorders and, 15, **16**
insomnia and, 40
Sleepwalking, **165,** 167–168, 173
Snoring, and sleep apnea, 83
Social factors, and shift work-related sleep, 209
Social withdrawal, and delayed sleep phase type of circadian rhythm disorder, 193
Sodium oxybate (GHB), and excessive daytime sleepiness, 122, 123
Statins, and insomnia, **39**
Stimulants
delayed sleep phase type of circadian rhythm disorder and, 197–198
excessive daytime sleepiness and, 120, **121,** 122
insomnia and, **39**
Stimulus control therapy, for insomnia, 43, **44,** 47–48
Stress, and sleepwalking, 168
Stroke
insomnia and, **38**
sleep apnea and, **85**
Structured activity, and circadian rhythm disorders, **192**
Stupor. *See* Idiopathic recurring stupor
Substance abuse. *See also* Alcohol use
benzodiazepines and, 56, 64
insomnia and, **39,** 40
Suggested Immobilization Test (SIT), and restless legs syndrome, 141, **142, 145**

sleep drive and increasing
duration of, **12**
types of disorders of, 19–20
Weight loss, and sleep apnea, 91
Willis, Sir Thomas, 139, 151
Women
menopause and risk of sleep
apnea in, 81
nightmare disorder and, 178
restless legs syndrome and, 145
Work. *See* Shift work type, of
circadian rhythm disorder, 206

Zaleplon
pharmacokinetics of, **52**
tolerance and efficacy of for
insomnia, 55
Zeitgebers, and circadian rhythms,
4
Zolpidem
efficacy of, for insomnia, 53, 55, 56
jet lag syndrome and, 211
parasomnias and, 171, **174**
pharmacokinetics of, **52**
trazodone compared to, 57